Quality Assessment Guidebook

A guide to assessing health services for adolescent clients

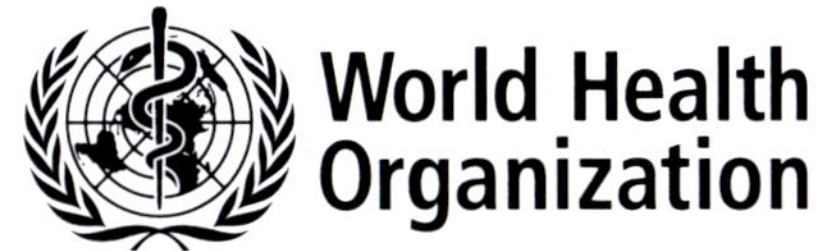

Acknowledgements

Several people contributed to the development of this guidebook. First, Siobhan Peattie gathered the tools to assess adolescent/youth-friendly health services that were available and in use. These tools included items developed by international organizations and initiatives, such as Engender Health, FOCUS on Young Adults, International Planned Parenthood Federation, Pathfinder International, Population Council and WHO, as well as those developed for use in specific countries, including the Brook Centre (United Kingdom of Great Britain and Northern Ireland), the National Adolescent-Friendly Clinic Initiative (South Africa) and the National Family Planning Council (Zimbabwe). Second, informed by already existing tools, Susanne Bantel drafted a bank of measurement tools to assess the WHO-listed characteristics of adolescent-friendly health services. Third, Korin Shrum built on this work to prepare a revised and expanded bank of measurement tools. Kristin Mmari honed the list of characteristics; reviewed and revised the assessment tools; prepared a framework to analyse data gathered through the assessment tools; and prepared a user guide. The guidebook was developed further as it was being used. As the development work evolved, draft tools were adapted and applied in several countries during research, notably in the Russian Federation, Mongolia and India, and during rapid assessment, notably in Kenya and Indonesia. This evolution led to a longer development process but one that was strengthened greatly by ongoing reality testing.

Several current and former staff members from WHO's Department of Child and Adolescent Health and Development contributed to the creation of this guidebook. They include (in alphabetical order) Paul Bloem, Krishna Bose, Susanne Carai, Jane Ferguson, Mathew Hodge and Varja Lipovsek. Venkatraman Chandra-Mouli oversaw development from the conceptual stage to the finished product.

Editing, design and layout by Inís Communication: www.iniscommunication.com

The illustrations in the guidebook have been prepared by Graham Ogilvie: graham@ogilviedesign.co.uk

Abbreviated terms

AFHS	adolescent-friendly health services
HIV	human immunodeficiency virus
RTI	respiratory tract infection
STI	sexually transmitted infection
WHO	World Health Organization

Contents

Introduction

1

Over the past few decades and throughout the world, the landscape of adolescent health has been altered dramatically. Currently, the total population of adolescents between the ages of 10 and 19 years is 1.2 billion – the largest generation of young people in history. The vast majority of adolescents (85%) live in developing countries where, in many areas, they make up more than a third of the population. They face a variety of different experiences given the diverse political, economic, social and cultural realities within their communities. Although, for many, adolescence is a period of learning and building confidence in a nurturing environment, for others it is a period of heightened risk and complex challenges.

Because more adolescents currently are reaching puberty earlier and marrying later, they face a longer period of sexual maturity before marriage and thus are more susceptible to a wider variety of reproductive health problems. Sexual activity during adolescence (within or outside marriage) puts adolescents at risk of sexual and reproductive health problems. These include early pregnancy (intended or otherwise), unsafe abortion, sexually transmitted infections including HIV, and sexual coercion and violence.[1] For many of these sexually active adolescents, reproductive health services, such as provision of contraception and treatment for sexually transmitted infections, either are not available or are provided in a way that makes adolescents feel unwelcome and embarrassed. As a result, adolescents are more likely to rely on resources outside the formal health-service provision system, such as home remedies, traditional methods of contraception, clandestine abortion or medicines from shops or traditional health practitioners. To address these issues, a number of initiatives have been developed and implemented that have made it easier for adolescents to obtain the good-quality health services that they need, in other words to make health services "adolescent-friendly".

To be considered adolescent-friendly, services should have the following characteristics.

EQUITABLE: All adolescents, not just certain groups, are able to obtain the health services they need.

ACCESSIBLE: Adolescents are able to obtain the services that are provided.

ACCEPTABLE: Health services are provided in ways that meet the expectations of adolescent clients.

APPROPRIATE: The health services that adolescents need are provided.

EFFECTIVE: The right health services are provided in the right way and make a positive contribution to the health of adolescents.

Below is a detailed list of adolescent-friendly characteristics that could contribute to making health facilities and other points of health service delivery more adolescent-friendly. They are organized according to the five broad dimensions of quality listed above. This list was created from a longer list of characteristics developed at the WHO Global Consultation in 2001[2] and in subsequent discussions. It has been further revised based on the outcomes of a systematic review of the published evidence in 2006.[3]

---

1 World Health Organization, Reproductive Health and Research and Child and Adolescent Health and Development departments. *Policy brief 4 – Implementing the reproductive health strategy*. Geneva, World Health Organization, 2006.

2 World Health Organization, Department of Child and Adolescent Health and Development. *Global consultation on adolescent friendly health services: a consensus statement, Geneva, 7–9 March 2001* (WHO/FCH/CAH/02.18). Geneva, World Health Organization, 2002.

3 Ross D, Dick B, Ferguson J, eds. *Preventing HIV in young people: a systematic review of the evidence from developing countries*. World Health Organization and Inter Agency Task Team on HIV and young people, 2006.

ADOLESCENT-FRIENDLY CHARACTERISTICS	
EQUITABLE: All adolescents, not just certain groups, are able to obtain the health services they need	
Characteristic	**Definition**
Policies and procedures are in place that do not restrict the provision of health services on any terms.	No policies or procedures restrict the provision of health services to adolescents on the basis of age, sex, social status, cultural background, ethnic origin, disability or any other area of difference.
Health-care providers treat all adolescent clients with equal care and respect, regardless of status.	Health-care providers administer the same level of care and consideration to all adolescents regardless of age, sex, social status, cultural background, ethnic origin, disability or any other reason.
Support staff treat all adolescent clients with equal care and respect, regardless of status.	Support staff administer the same level of care and consideration to all adolescents regardless of age, sex, social status, cultural background, ethnic origin, disability or any other reason.
ACCESSIBLE: Adolescents are able to obtain the health services that are provided	
Characteristic	**Definition**
Policies and procedures are in place that ensure that health services are either free or affordable to adolescents.	All adolescents are able to receive health services free of charge or are able to afford any charges that might be in place.
The point of health service delivery has convenient hours of operation.	Health services are available to all adolescents during convenient times of the day.
Adolescents are well-informed about the range of available reproductive health services and how to obtain them.	Adolescents are aware of what health services are being provided, where they are provided and how to obtain them.
Community members understand the benefits that adolescents will gain by obtaining the health services they need, and support their provision.	Community members (including parents) are well-informed about how the provision of health services could help adolescents. They support the provision of these services as well as their use by adolescents.
Some health services and health-related commodities are provided to adolescents in the community by selected community members, outreach workers and adolescents themselves.	Efforts are under way to provide health services close to where adolescents are. Depending on the situation, outreach workers, selected community members (e.g. sports coaches) and adolescents themselves may be involved in this.
ACCEPTABLE: Health services are provided in ways that meet the expectations of adolescent clients	
Characteristic	**Definition**
Policies and procedures are in place that guarantee client confidentiality.	Policies and procedures are in place that maintain adolescents' confidentiality at all times (except where staff are obliged by legal requirements to report incidents such as sexual assaults, road traffic accidents or gunshot wounds, to the relevant authorities). Policies and procedures address: – registration – information on the identity of the adolescent and the presenting issue are gathered in confidence; – consultation – confidentiality is maintained throughout the visit of the adolescent to the point of health service delivery (i.e. before, during and after a consultation); – record-keeping – case-records are kept in a secure place, accessible only to authorized personnel; – disclosure of information – staff do not disclose any information given to or received from an adolescent to third parties such as family members, school teachers or employers, without the adolescent's consent.

Continues...

Continued from previous page

Characteristic	Definition
The point of health service delivery ensures privacy.	The point of health service delivery is located in a place that ensures the privacy of adolescent users. It has a layout that is designed to ensure privacy throughout an adolescent's visit. This includes the point of entry, the reception area, the waiting area, the examination area and the patient-record storage area.
Health-care providers are non-judgmental, considerate, and easy to relate to.	Health-care providers do not criticize their adolescent patients even if they do not approve of the patients' words and actions. They are considerate to their patients and reach out to them in a friendly manner.
The point of health service delivery ensures consultations occur in a short waiting time, with or without an appointment, and (where necessary) swift referral.	Adolescents are able to consult with health-care providers at short notice, whether or not they have a formal appointment. If their medical condition is such that they need to be referred elsewhere, the referral appointment also takes place within a short time frame.
The point of health service delivery has an appealing and clean environment.	A point of health service delivery that is welcoming, attractive and clean.
The point of health service delivery provides information and education through a variety of channels.	Information that is relevant to the health of adolescents is available in different formats (e.g. posters, booklets and leaflets). Materials are presented in a familiar language, easy to understand and eye-catching.
Adolescents are actively involved in designing, assessing and providing health services.	Adolescents are given the opportunity to share their experiences in obtaining health services and to express their needs and preferences. They are involved in certain appropriate aspects of health-service provision.
APPROPRIATE: The health services that adolescents need are provided	
Characteristic	**Definition**
The required package of health care is provided to fulfil the needs of all adolescents either at the point of health service delivery or through referral linkages.	The health needs and problems of all adolescents are addressed by the health services provided at the point of health service delivery or through referral linkages. The services provided meet the special needs of marginalized groups of adolescents and those of the majority.
EFFECTIVE: The right health services are provided in the right way and make a positive contribution to the health of adolescents	
Characteristic	**Definition**
Health-care providers have the required competencies to work with adolescents and to provide them with the required health services.	Health-care providers have the required knowledge and skills to work with adolescents and to provide them with the required health services.
Health-care providers use evidence-based protocols and guidelines to provide health services.	Health service provision is based on protocols and guidelines that are technically sound and of proven usefulness. Ideally, they should be adapted to the requirements of the local situation and approved by the relevant authorities.
Health-care providers are able to dedicate sufficient time to work effectively with their adolescent clients.	Health-care providers are able to dedicate sufficient time to work effectively with their adolescent clients.
The point of health service delivery has the required equipment, supplies, and basic services necessary to deliver the required health services.	Each point of health service delivery has the necessary equipment, supplies, including medicines, and basic services (e.g. water and sanitation) needed to deliver the health services.

Purpose of the Quality Assessment Guidebook

This guidebook is designed to assist national and district health managers, as well as managers and staff at health facilities[4], to assess the quality of their services for adolescents and young people in relation to the list of adolescent-friendly characteristics. This assessment will help managers and staff identify where their services and systems are already "adolescent-friendly" and will suggest where and how improvements can be made.

4 The term "point of health service delivery" is used in the characteristics, however from here on the term "health facility" will be used. The same methods and tools could be used in assessing the provision of health services and commodities (e.g. in pharmacies, clinics set up in places of work and education etc.).

How to use the Quality Assessment Guidebook

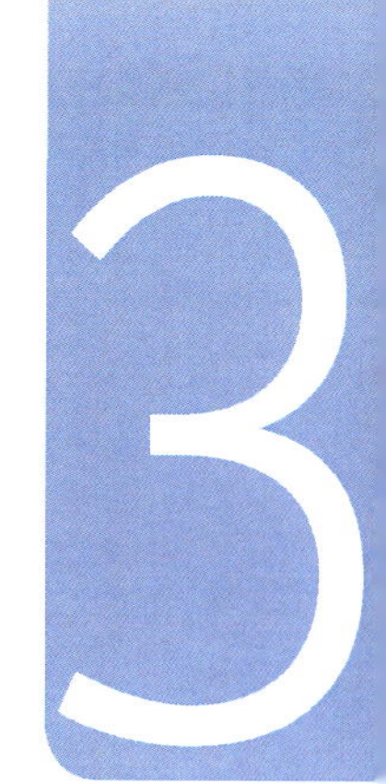

a. Pre-planning for the assessment

A number of decisions must be made before an assessment of the adolescent-friendliness of health services can be conducted. To help you get started, below is a list of questions you should consider before you start planning the assessment:

1) What is the scope of your assessment?

a. How many health facilities will be assessed?

b. What is the size of the health facility?
   i. How many health-care providers are employed at the facility?
   ii. Is there an outreach component?
   iii. What types of health services does the health facility offer?
   iv. Will all the types of health services be assessed or only those relating to reproductive health?

c. Will all the adolescent-friendly health characteristics be assessed or is the focus to be on assessing a subset or a particular domain (e.g. looking at the characteristics that deal with health-care providers)?

2) Have national quality standards been developed by the Ministry of Health?

If so, the assessment should be based on characteristics of adolescent-friendly health services that are most closely aligned with the established standards. As an example, one of the standards agreed upon by the Ministry of Health in Tanzania is that "service providers in all delivery points have the required knowledge, skills and positive attitudes to provide sexual and reproductive health services to adolescents effectively and in a friendly manner". This standard could be aligned with the following characteristics.

a. Characteristic 11: Health-care providers are non-judgmental, considerate, and easy to relate to.

b. Characteristic 17: Health-care providers have the required competencies to work with adolescents and to provide them with the required health services.

c. Characteristic 18: Health-care providers use evidence-based protocols and guidelines to provide health services.

The assessment then could serve as a mechanism for tracking how standards are reached. If some standards cannot be linked to one of the 20 characteristics of adolescent-friendly health services, additional questions and/or observation items should be framed.

3) What time and resources are available?

a. How many days can you and your team work on the assessment?

b. Do you need extra funds to help you carry out this assessment?

c. Are adolescents able to be involved in this assessment?

d. Are community members (e.g. parents) able to be involved in this assessment?

These questions are important because they greatly influence the type of data you will collect and the preparations that you must make to plan and strategize your assessment.

Example of pre-planning for the assessment

In the (fictional) rural district of Boyumangu, there are five health facilities and one hospital. Although the district health manager would like to assess these facilities on all of the characteristics of adolescent-friendly health services, she knows that she does not have a great deal of time and money. Instead, she decides to assess a subset of the list of characteristics and concentrate only on assessing the health-care providers of the health facilities and hospital that provide reproductive health services. With this in mind, she selects the following list of adolescent-friendly characteristics.

- Health-care providers treat all adolescent clients with equal care and respect, regardless of status.
- Health-care providers are non-judgmental, considerate and easy to relate to.
- Health-care providers have the required competencies to work with adolescents.
- Health-care providers use evidence-based protocols and guidelines to provide health services.
- Health-care providers are able to dedicate sufficient time to work effectively with their adolescent clients.

From this list, she knows that she must collect data from adolescent clients and the health-care providers from each of the health centres. She also wants to observe the interactions of a small sample of health-care providers and their adolescent clients. She decides that planning, collecting and analysing the data for this assessment will take approximately two to three weeks. From this initial appraisal, she can start to assemble her team and set up a meeting to plan the assessment.

b. Planning for the assessment

The assessment team:

Depending on the scope of your assessment and the time and resources you have available, your first activity is to identify your assessment team. Ideally, the assessment team should consist of a member of the district health management team, health facility manager(s), adolescents and respected members of the community (e.g. parents of youth, teachers and community leaders). The member of the district health management team could be a team leader and coordinate the implementation of the assessment.

Certain personal characteristics and qualities are important when collecting information from others. In selecting people to be included in the assessment team, you should choose those who have some of the necessary skills and/or experience, summarized in the following box:

Useful qualities of assessment team members

- Good listening abilities: patient and willing to listen and learn from people.
- Good communication abilities; able to manage a discussion; knowledgeable in local languages, where necessary.
- Culturally sensitive: aware and respectful of local customs, norms and beliefs.
- Knowledgeable about issues related to sexual and reproductive health and comfortable talking about them.
- Experience in working with young people.
- Respectful and non-judgmental attitudes towards young people.
- Experience of working with young people and community members

Preparing the team:

Once the team has been selected, all members should be briefed fully about the concept of adolescent-friendly health services and given an overview of the assessment before it begins. The best way to do this is to hold a meeting during which the team can discuss the following:

- the meaning of "adolescent-friendly" health services
- the list of adolescent-friendly service characteristics
- an overview of the Adolescent-Friendly Health Services Quality Assessment Guidebook
- the aims and overview of the data collection process
- the workplan, which should be developed during the meeting
- the roles and responsibilities of team members.

Developing a workplan for the assessment:

It is essential to develop a workplan for the assessment process to ensure that all steps are taken and to identify all the resources needed to carry out the assessment. Ideally, the whole assessment team should be involved in developing the workplan. This means that everyone should have a clear and common understanding of the assessment and their roles and responsibilities. The plan should be completed before the beginning of data collection, although it can and should be modified where necessary, as it is very common to encounter unexpected changes that can affect the workplan.

The following page contains an example of a workplan. Notice that it includes a list of the necessary activities, the desired outputs of each activity, the persons responsible and the resources needed to accomplish the activity.

Example of a workplan for assessment

Activity	What is the expected output of this activity?	Who is responsible for this activity?	Who else will be involved?	What resources will be needed (e.g. transport, materials, money)?	Where will this activity take place?	What are the start and end dates of this task?		✓
						Start	End	
1. Form team	Team	District health manager	District health team and selected health facility managers	None	District centre	6 March	8 March	
2. Meet with team to introduce process and select sites	Five to six health facilities identified	District health manager	All team members	None	District health meeting room	10 March	10 March	
3. Prepare briefing workshop	Logistical and other preparations for workshop completed	District health manager	None	Copies of the Adolescent-Friendly Health Services Quality Assessment Guidebook, flipchart paper, marker pens, notepads, pens	District centre	13 March	14 March	
4. Hold workshop to brief team	Team members understand process and roles; workplan developed	District health manager	All team members	Refreshments	District health meeting room	15 March	15 March	
5. Data collection meeting	Logistical and other preparations planned for collecting data	Team members		Refreshments	District centre	16 March	16 March	
6. Pretest data collection instruments	A final set of data collection instruments	District health manager	Team members	Transport, data collection instruments, notepads, pens	Sites 1–6	19 March	20 March	

Activity	What is the expected output of this activity?	Who is responsible for this activity?	Who else will be involved?	What resources will be needed (e.g. transport, materials, money)?	Where will this activity take place?	What are the start and end dates of this task?		✓
						Start	End	
7. Carry out data collection at selected sites: – adolescent client tool among 10 adolescent clients per site – health-care provider tool among three health-care providers per site – one focus group among adolescents in community per site – one observation among selected characteristics per site	Data collected on all essential adolescent-friendly characteristics	District health manager	Team members	Transport, data collection instruments	Sites 1–6	21 March	4 April	
8. Analyze findings and compile synthesis report	Findings from various consultation meetings shared, compiled, and discussed	District health manager	All team members	Flipchart paper, marker pens, computer, paper	District centre	5 April	12 April	
9. Present findings to district health team and others	Findings and conclusions shared with others to start planning process	District health manager	Other team members	Flipchart paper, marker pens	District health meeting room	14 April	14 April	

Data collection:

The step after debriefing the team and developing a preliminary workplan is deciding how data will be collected for the assessment.

There are eight data collection instruments for assessing the list of adolescent-friendly characteristics:

- Adolescent client tool
- Health-care provider tool
- Support staff tool
- Health facility manager tool
- Outreach worker tool
- Community member tool
- Adolescent-in-community tool[5]
- Observation guide.

Below is a table of the adolescent-friendly characteristics and their corresponding data collection instruments:

Characteristic	AC	HP	SS	M	OW	CM	A in C	OG
Policies and procedures are in place that do not restrict the provision of health services on any terms	✓	✓		✓			✓	
Health-care providers treat all adolescent clients with equal care and respect, regardless of status.	✓	✓					✓	
Support staff treat all adolescent clients with equal care and respect, regardless of status	✓		✓				✓	
Policies and procedures are in place that ensure that health services are either free or affordable to adolescents	✓			✓			✓	
The point of health service delivery has convenient hours of operation	✓			✓			✓	
Adolescents are well-informed about the range of available reproductive health services and how to obtain them	✓						✓	
Community members understand the benefits that adolescents will gain by obtaining the health services they need, and support their provision	✓	✓				✓	✓	
Some health services and health-related commodities are provided to adolescents in the community by selected community members, outreach workers and adolescents themselves	✓			✓	✓		✓	

Continues...

5 This tool assesses adolescents who are contacted in the vicinity of, but not in, the health facility; they may or may not have been to the health facility being assessed.

Continued from previous page

Characteristic	AC	HP	SS	M	OW	CM	A in C	OG
Policies and procedures are in place that guarantee client confidentiality	✓	✓		✓				✓
The point of health service delivery ensures privacy	✓	✓		✓				✓
Health-care providers are non-judgmental, considerate, and easy to relate to	✓							✓
The point of health service delivery ensures consultations occur in a short waiting time, with or without an appointment, and (where necessary) swift referral	✓	✓	✓					✓
The point of health service delivery has an appealing and clean environment	✓							✓
The point of health service delivery provides information and education through a variety of channels	✓			✓				✓
Adolescents are actively involved in designing, assessing and providing health services	✓			✓				
The required package of health care is provided to fulfil the needs of all adolescents either at the point of health service delivery or through referral linkages	✓	✓		✓				
Health-care providers have the required competencies to work with adolescents and to provide them with the required health services.	✓	✓		✓				✓
Health-care providers use evidence-based protocols and guidelines to provide health services		✓		✓				✓
Health-care providers are able to dedicate sufficient time to work effectively with their adolescent clients	✓	✓						
The point of health service delivery has the required equipment, supplies, and basic services necessary to deliver the required health services	✓	✓		✓				✓

Key: AC = adolescent client tool; A in C = adolescent-in-community tool; CM = community member tool; HP = health-care provider tool; M = health facility manager tool; OG = observation guide; OW = outreach worker tool; SS = support staff tool.

Note that the only data collection instrument that is used for nearly every characteristic is the adolescent client tool. Although collecting data from adolescent clients is obviously a key source of information for the assessment, it is important to realize that adolescents will not be aware of all that is required to provide them with quality health services. In addition, the views of adolescent clients represent one type of perspective of how the services are delivered. For these reasons, it is important to use more than just the adolescent client tool to collect data on each characteristic. Although it may not be feasible to use all the recommended data collection instruments for each characteristic, at least two different sources of information are important for strengthening the validity of the data you collect. Reviewing all data collection instruments before making this decision will save considerable time.

Once the team decides on the type of data that will be collected for each characteristic, the next step is to review the data collection instruments that will be used. Keep in mind that most of these instruments will need to be translated and back-translated from English into the local language of the area in which the assessment will take place.

Tips on translating and back-translating instruments

A new approach for ensuring that data collection instruments are *reliable, complete, accurate* and *culturally appropriate* when translated from a source language to a target language is called "the committee approach".

What is the committee approach?

The committee approach involves convening a group of people who have complementary skills and assigning them specific roles. The committee includes several translators, at least one "referee", translation reviewers and someone with knowledge about designing questions. Several translators independently translate the instrument from the source language to the target language. A meeting is then held with the translators, the translation reviewers and other members of the assessment team, to discuss the translated versions of the instrument. From this meeting, a revised version of the translated instrument is produced, which then goes to the referees or "judges" who make the final decisions. In this case, the referee or judge could be the assessment team leader. The data collection instrument is then pretested (see below).

When is the translation deemed reliable?

When the translated text conveys the intended meaning of the original text.

When is the translation complete?

When the translated text does not add any new information and does not omit any information provided in the source document.

When is the translation accurate?

When the translation is free of spelling and grammatical errors.

When is the translation culturally appropriate?

When the message conveyed in the translated text is appropriate for the target population.

Adapted from: Pan Y, de la Puente M. *Census Bureau guideline for the translation of data collection instruments and supporting materials: criteria for achieving a good translation and the translation of surveys. Documentation on how the guideline was developed* http://www.census.gov/srd/papers/pdf/rsm2005-06.pdf, accessed 17 June 2008.

Pretesting the instruments

After the data collection instruments have been translated and/or adapted to the cultural context, each also must be pretested among a similar group of informants. A pretest of the adolescent client tool, for example, will need to be conducted among a small sample of approximately 3–5 adolescent clients. Pretesting allows you to determine whether the data collection instruments will work in the way that is intended. You can consider the pretest a "trial run" of the instruments where you can uncover any defects in the questions. After pretesting, you should expect to make some changes to the format or content of the data collection instrument. For this reason, it is important to remember the first rule of pretesting: do not pretest with a final, printed version of your data collection instrument.

Guidelines on pretesting:

1) The first stage of the pretest process is to make sure that all participants are aware that they are taking a pretest. You can simply tell them that you are testing to see whether the questions that are going to be asked in the assessment make sense to them.

2) Remember that the pretest participants are the experts when it comes to understanding your questions, but you are the ultimate authority. There may be times when suggestions made by the participants are impractical or not easily understood.

3) Note how many times a participant answers, "I don't know". Too many of these responses may indicate that the question should be reworded.

4) Note how long it takes to conduct the interview. Interviews that are too long may need to be shortened, especially for use among adolescents.

5) At the end of the interview or after the data collection instrument has been completed, ask participants to comment on the questions and on whether additional questions relevant to the assessment are needed. Because people are often reluctant to admit difficulty in responding, ask whether they believe other people would have difficulty and which questions might pose problems.

Remember, each data collection instrument must be pretested. It also is of first importance, after you have collected useful comments from pretest participants, to go back and revise the instruments based on these comments.

c. Data collection

The sample frame for the data collection activities:

Below is a table that lists the recommended number of respondents for each data collection instrument. Note, however, that this number greatly depends upon the scope of your assessment and the resources that you have available.

Data collection instrument	Recommended sample frame
Adolescent client tool	Approximately six adolescents per health facility; can be divided into three male adolescents and three female adolescents, but this depends on the type of service being assessed e.g. antenatal clinic or STI clinic.
Health-care provider tool	In facilities where there are fewer than five health-care providers, all should be interviewed; where there are more than five but fewer than 10 health-care providers, at least five should be interviewed; where there are more than 10 health-care providers, 50% should be interviewed.
Support staff tool	At each facility, the primary support staff member is usually the receptionist. It might be worthwhile to ask which other staff are most likely to come in contact with the most adolescents. In general, approximately three support staff per health facility should be interviewed.
Health facility manager tool	Typically, there is one manager per health facility. Each manager should be interviewed.
Outreach worker tool	Depending on the size of the community and the number and types of outreach workers, a general recommendation is to interview at least five per community.
Community member tool	Community members can consist of husbands of young women, mothers-in-law, parents of adolescents, teachers of adolescent students and other community leaders. The selection of community members will depend greatly on the cultural context. In most cases, parents should be the primary informant, as they are likely to exert the most influence on whether adolescents seek care at the health facility. When thinking about selecting a sample, try to include various types of people from the community so that you can obtain a wide range of viewpoints. When selecting parents to interview, for example, make sure that you speak to mothers and fathers from different socioeconomic groups. In general, choose two to three people from each category (e.g. mothers, fathers, religious leaders, teachers).
Adolescent-in-community tool	A focus-group discussion could be conducted among eight to 10 adolescents in a community. Otherwise, approximately five to six adolescents could be interviewed separately in a community.
Observation guide	If you are going to be assessing Characteristic 17 "Health-care providers have the required competencies to work with adolescents and to provide them with the required health services.", you must observe approximately three to five interactions between health-care providers and adolescent clients per site. The other characteristics that require observations are more general to the health facility.

The two main methods that you will use for collecting information for the assessment are individual interviews and focus-group discussions. Individual interviews are semi-structured discussions with an individual key informant, following a question guide. Focus-group discussions are held with a group of about 8 to 10 individuals of similar characteristics (e.g. mothers of adolescents), and are loosely guided by a list of topics.

For both individual interviews and focus-group discussions there are some guiding rules that should always be applied when collecting information:

1) At the start of any interview you should explain the purpose for talking to them, what the procedures will be for the interview and approximately how long the interview will take.

2) It is important to discuss confidentiality with the interviewees (i.e. how will you ensure that no one else knows about this interview or the information they provided to you) as well as the risks and benefits of participating in the interview.

3) All information provided in the discussion should be recorded, either by taking notes or by using a tape-recorder during the interview.

4) Facilitators of focus-group discussions or interviewers for the individual interviews should be chosen with care to make sure that cultural or social barriers do not hinder the discussion. It is recommended to use female interviewers for female informants, for example, especially if the topic

of interest is reproductive health. Health workers also should not interview people who attend the health facility where they themselves work, as this would likely inhibit critical and honest comments about the services.

5) The place of the interview or focus-group discussion should be chosen with care. The venue should be neutral; for example, focus-group discussions with adolescents should not be held at the health centre about which they will answer questions. The venue also should ensure privacy so that the interview cannot be overheard by others.

6) At the end of the interview, the interviewer or facilitator should thank the participants for their time and information and should notify them about how they will find out about the results of this study.

For a complete set of data collection tools for this assessment, please see Section 5.

d. Scoring and summarizing the data

An efficient way to summarize all the data that has been collected is to calculate a score for each adolescent-friendly health characteristic that was assessed. A score is calculated by quantifying the information collected from each data source. On the score sheet, each question has a number that corresponds to the question number found in the relevant data collection instrument. Scoring is based on a points system according to the number of questions that were asked from each data source, as well as the number of data sources used. Low points are assigned for lower quality performance and high points are assigned for stronger performance or higher quality. An overall score for each characteristic is calculated by averaging all of the scores from each data source. The overall scores will give you a general sense of how well the facility performs on the characteristic being measured and will help you to track improvements over time. See the following scoring sheets created for each adolescent-friendly health characteristic.

e. Presenting the data

Once the data have been summarized and characteristics have been scored, the next stage involves presenting the findings to others so that they can be verified and discussed to help plan for the future. There are two main audience groups to whom the findings should be presented.

- Community members and others who provided the information for the assessment. The purpose of sharing the findings with this group is to provide them with feedback on the process with which they were involved and to check that the analysis and conclusions made by the assessment team accurately reflect the situation in the community. The findings should be presented to community members in an appropriate format, such as a community meeting, with sufficient time allotted for feedback from the audience. It also may be appropriate to hold separate meetings among adolescents, health-care providers and parents of adolescents.
- Decision-makers, including the entire district health team and other institutions and organizations that were involved in the assessment. The findings should be presented to this group in a planning meeting, which will serve as a starting-point for discussing and resolving gaps in health service provision and barriers to access by adolescents.

In both cases, the findings should include statements about the strengths and weaknesses of the health facilities that were assessed and recommendations for improvement. Charts could be developed and distributed to members of the audience on some of the more detailed findings, such as the information shown in the following table:

AFHS characteristic	Findings	Source(s)	Comments
The point of health service delivery ensures privacy	Interruptions frequently occur while a provider and client are in the examination room.	Health-care providers and adolescent clients	– There should be agreement on the need to avoid interrupting a health-care provider when he/she is with a client, unless there are pressing circumstances. – All staff need to be made aware of this agreement and be encouraged to follow it.

AFHS = adolescent-friendly health services.

When making a presentation of the findings to the different audience groups, overhead slides or PowerPoint slides should be developed for the following points.

- Purpose and aims of the assessment – why you decided to conduct it.
- Overview of the process – what did you want to assess? Who did you collect the information from? How did you do it?
- Methods and tools used – what type of data collection did you conduct? How were the data collection instruments developed?
- Results of the assessment – what were the most important findings from the assessment? What were the different views from the different data sources?
- Conclusions and recommendations – what were the main conclusions? What are your recommendations for what should happen next?

f. Planning for improvements

Undertaking an assessment is the first step to improving or making the health services more adolescent-friendly and the data you collect can be used to develop an action plan for improving the quality of health services at your facility. Below is an example of a chart that can help you and your assessment team make improvements for each of the characteristics found to be weak (having scores of less than 50%) in the assessment.

Characteristic 1: Policies and procedures are in place that do not restrict the provision of health services on any terms

What needs to be done	Responsibility	Time frame for improvement	Needed inputs

g. Monitoring facilities over time

Assessment scores also can serve as baseline scores against which to monitor changes in the adolescent-friendly health characteristics over time. To monitor the facilities, you should undertake an assessment at various intervals; for example, after the first assessment you may want to improve the facilities over a six-month period. You may then undertake a follow-up assessment 18 months after the baseline assessment was conducted. The follow-up assessment should measure the same characteristics as in the first assessment and compare scores over time. Aspects of the health services that still need improvement also can be identified, and changes can be planned for the next strategic planning cycle.

Scoring sheets for data analysis

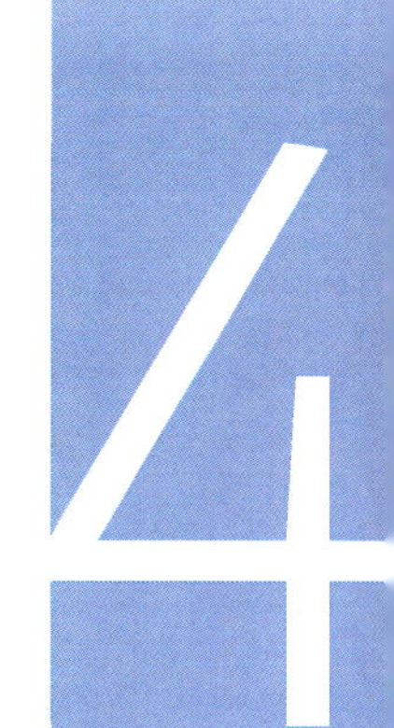

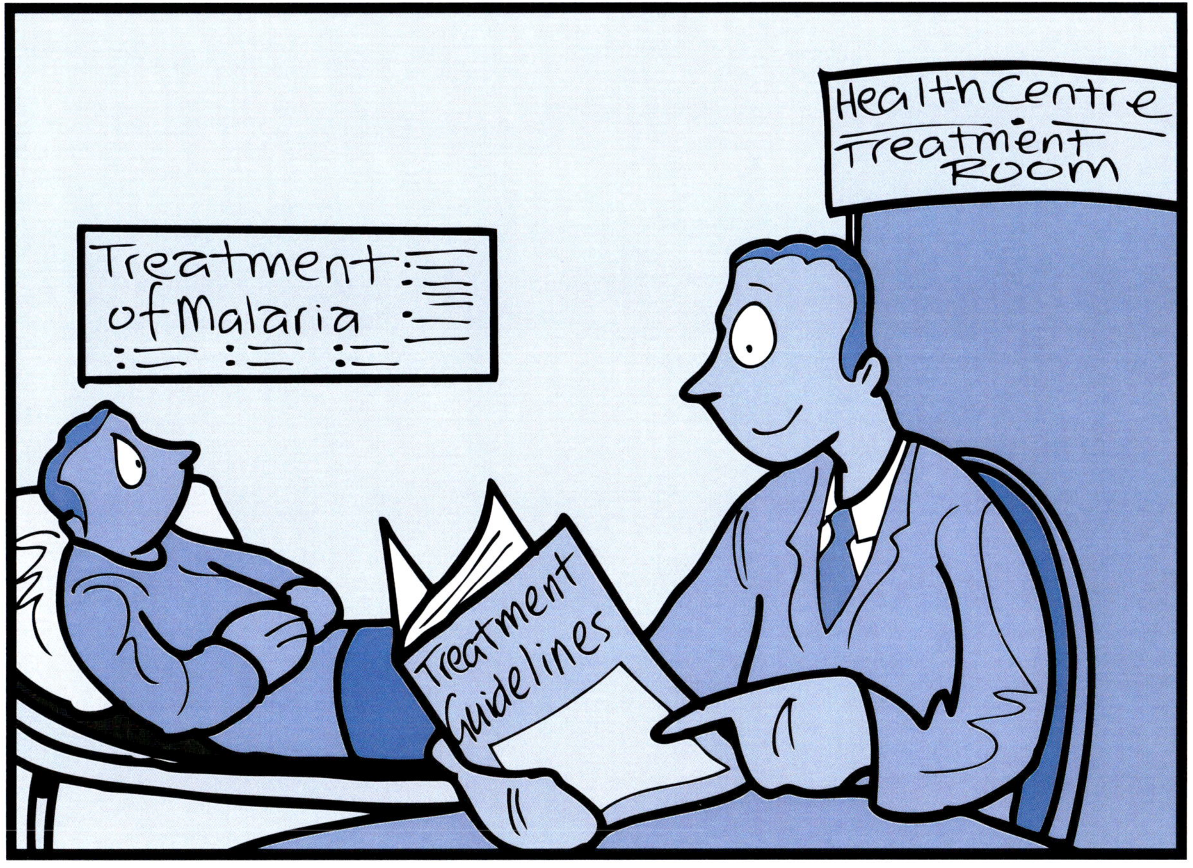

NB The column "No." refers to questions in the relevant interview tool.

No.	Question	Response	Score
6	Have you ever come to this health facility and not been able to receive a particular type of health service?	0=Yes, 1=No	Total "No" divided by total number of adolescent clients interviewed
7	Are any health services offered at this facility that you think some groups of adolescents might not be able to receive?	0=Yes, 1=No	Total "No" divided by total number of adolescent clients interviewed

See Section 5, "Instruments for data collection", for all questions.

CHARACTERISTIC 1

Policies and procedures are in place that do not restrict the provision of health services on any terms

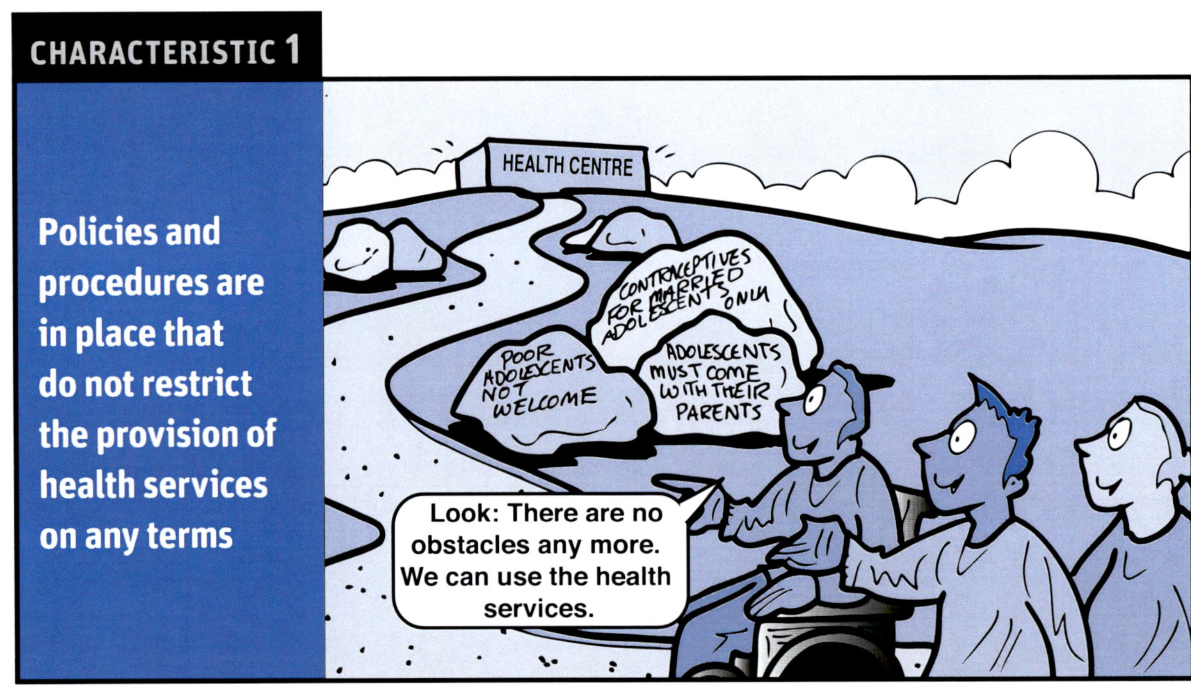

Adolescent client tool:

No.	Question	Response	Score
6	Have you ever come to this health facility and not been able to receive a particular type of health service?	0=Yes, 1=No	Total "No" divided by total number of adolescent clients interviewed
7	Are any health services offered at this facility that you think some groups of adolescents might not be able to receive?	0=Yes, 1=No	Total "No" divided by total number of adolescent clients interviewed
	Aggregate adolescent client score		**Total score**

Health-care provider tool:

No.	Question	Response	Score
5	Are there certain policies or procedures at this facility that might restrict the provision of health services to some groups of adolescents, such as those who are less than a certain age; those who are not married; or those who belong to a certain group, such as people living or working on the street?	0=Yes, 1=No	Total "No" divided by total number of health-care providers interviewed
	Aggregate health-care provider score		**Total score**

Manager tool:

No.	Question	Response	Score
3	Are there certain policies or procedures at this facility that might restrict the provision of health services to some adolescents, such as those who are less than a certain age; those who are not married; or those who belong to a certain group, such as people living or working on the street?	0=Yes, 1=No	Total "No" divided by total number of managers interviewed
	Aggregate manager score		**Total score**

Adolescent-in-community tool:

No.	Question	Response	Score
1	Have you or your friends been denied health services at the health facility (name of facility)?	0=Yes, 1=No	Total "No" divided by total number of adolescents in community interviewed
	Aggregate adolescent-in-community score		**Total score**

Overall score on Characteristic 1

	Category	Min – Max	Score
1	Aggregate adolescent client score	0 – 2	
2	Aggregate health-care provider score	0 – 1	
3	Aggregate manager score	0 – 1	
4	Aggregate adolescent-in-community score	0 – 1	
	Absolute total score	0 – 5	
	Relative score for Characteristic 1	0 to 100%	$\left(\frac{\text{Total score}}{5}\right) \times 100$

SCORING SHEETS

CHARACTERISTIC 2

Health-care providers treat all adolescent clients with equal care and respect, regardless of status

HEALTH CENTRE
I went there and the nurse and doctor treated me with respect.
WAITING ROOM
Really? Maybe I'll go too now.
Seeking help?

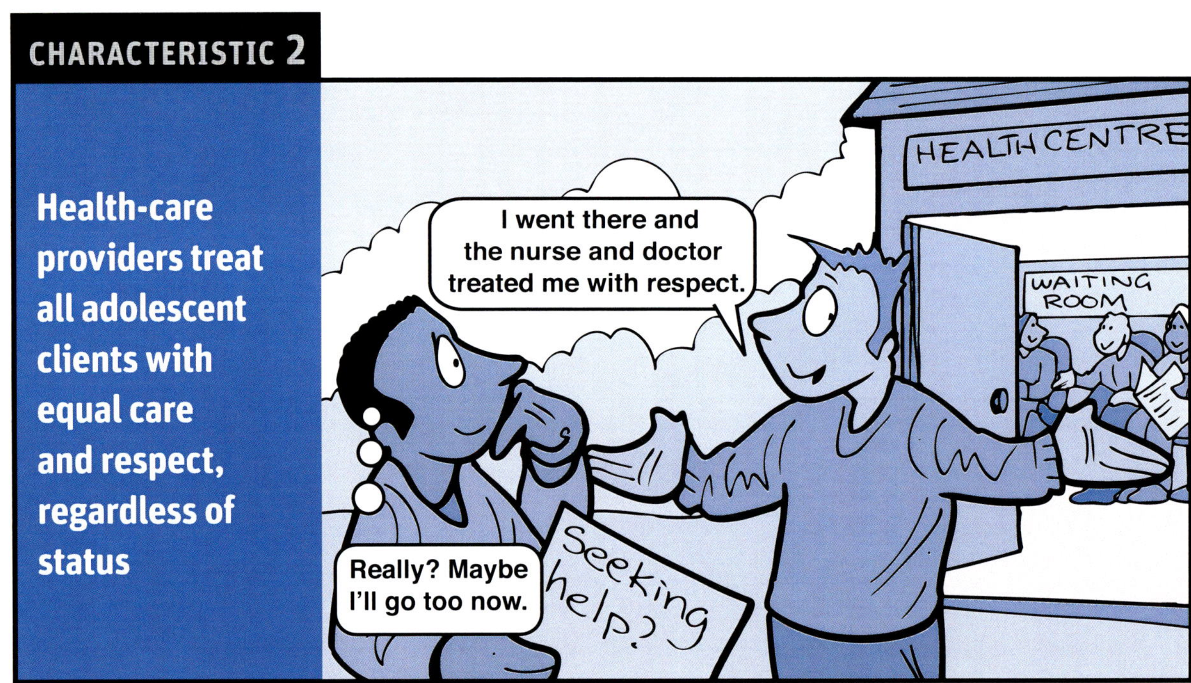

Adolescent client tool:

No.	Question	Response	Score
8	Has the health-care provider treated you in a manner that made you feel respected?	0=No, 1=Yes	Total "Yes" divided by total number of adolescent clients interviewed
9	Did the health-care provider make you feel comfortable?	0=No, 1=Yes	Total "Yes" divided by total number of adolescent clients interviewed
	Aggregate adolescent client score		**Total score**

Health-care provider tool:

No.	Question	Response	Score
7	Are there some groups of adolescents who you do not feel comfortable dealing with ?	0=Yes, 1=No	Total "No" divided by total number of health-care providers interviewed
	Aggregate health-care provider score		**Total score**

Adolescent-in-community tool:

No.	Question	Response (0=Yes, 1=No)	Score
2	Has a health-care provider at the facility treated you or your friends in a manner that made you feel upset?	0=Yes, 1=No	Total "No" divided by total number of adolescents in community interviewed
	Aggregate adolescent-in-community score		**Total score**

Overall score on Characteristic 2

	Category	Min – Max	Score
1	Aggregate adolescent client score	0 – 2	
2	Aggregate health-care provider score	0 – 1	
3	Aggregate adolescent-in-community score	0 – 1	
	Absolute total score	0 – 4	
	Relative score for Characteristic 2	0 to 100%	$\left(\frac{\text{Total score}}{4}\right) \times 100$

SCORING SHEETS

CHARACTERISTIC 3

Support staff treat all adolescent clients with equal care and respect, regardless of status

Health Centre
How are YOU?
Come in please and sit down. You don't look well. You can see a doctor soon.

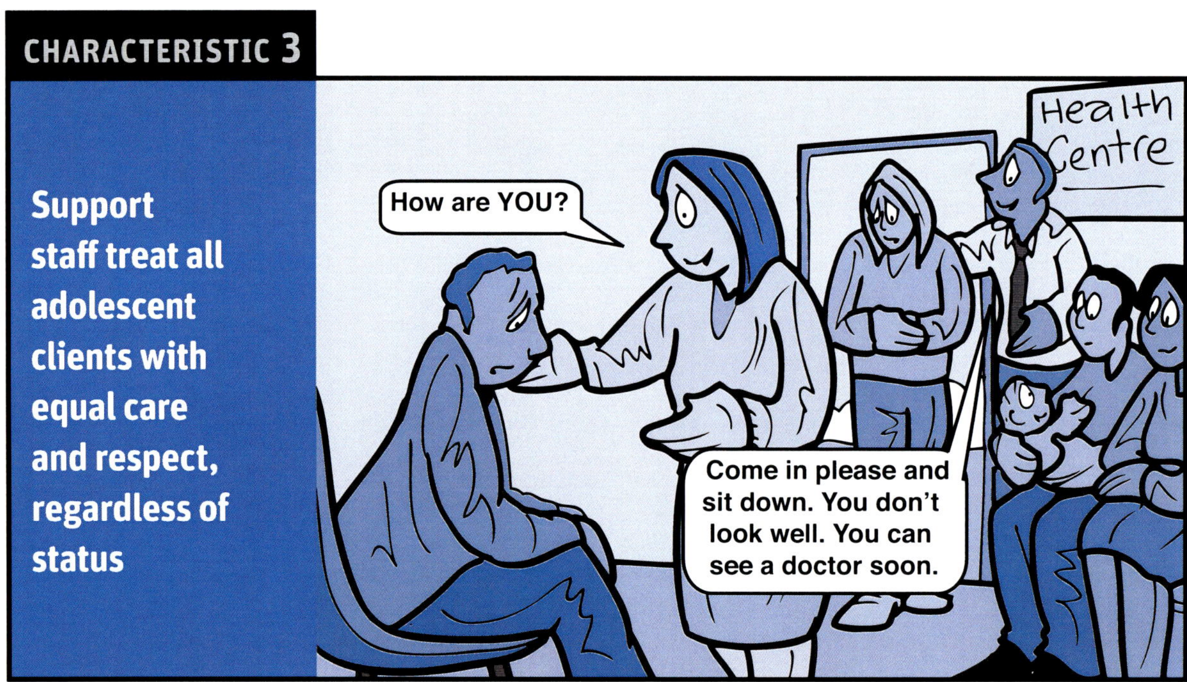

Adolescent client tool:

No.	Question	Response	Score
10	Has the receptionist treated you in a manner in which you would want to be treated?	0=No, 1=Yes	Total "Yes" divided by total number of adolescent clients interviewed
11	Did the receptionist make you feel comfortable?	0=No, 1=Yes	Total "Yes" divided by total number of adolescent clients interviewed
12	Have other support staff, such as security staff, clerical staff and cleaning staff, treated you in a manner in which you would want to be treated?	0=No, 1=Yes	Total "Yes" divided by total number of adolescent clients interviewed
13	Did other support staff, such as security staff, clerical staff and cleaning staff, make you feel comfortable?	0=No, 1=Yes	Total "Yes" divided by total number of adolescent clients interviewed
	Aggregate adolescent client score		**Total score**

Support staff tool:

No.	Question	Response	Score
5	Are there some groups of adolescents who you do not feel comfortable dealing with?	0=Yes, 1=No	Total "No" divided by total number of support staff interviewed
	Aggregate support staff score		**Total score**

Adolescent-in-community tool:

No.	Question	Response	Score
3	Has the receptionist or any other type of support staff treated you or your friends in a manner that made you feel upset?	0=Yes, 1=No	Total "No" divided by total number of adolescents in community interviewed
	Aggregate adolescent-in-community score		**Total score**

Overall score on Characteristic 3

	Category	Min – Max	Score
1	Aggregate adolescent client score	0 – 4	
2	Aggregate health-care provider score	0 – 1	
3	Aggregate adolescent-in-community score	0 – 1	
	Absolute total score	0 – 6	
	Relative score for Characteristic 3	0 to 100%	$\left(\frac{\text{Total score}}{6}\right) \times 100$

SCORING SHEETS

CHARACTERISTIC 4

Policies and procedures are in place that ensure that health services are either free or affordable to adolescents

Health Centre
Services Provided Free of charge
What a relief! I can get the health services I need without asking my parents for money.

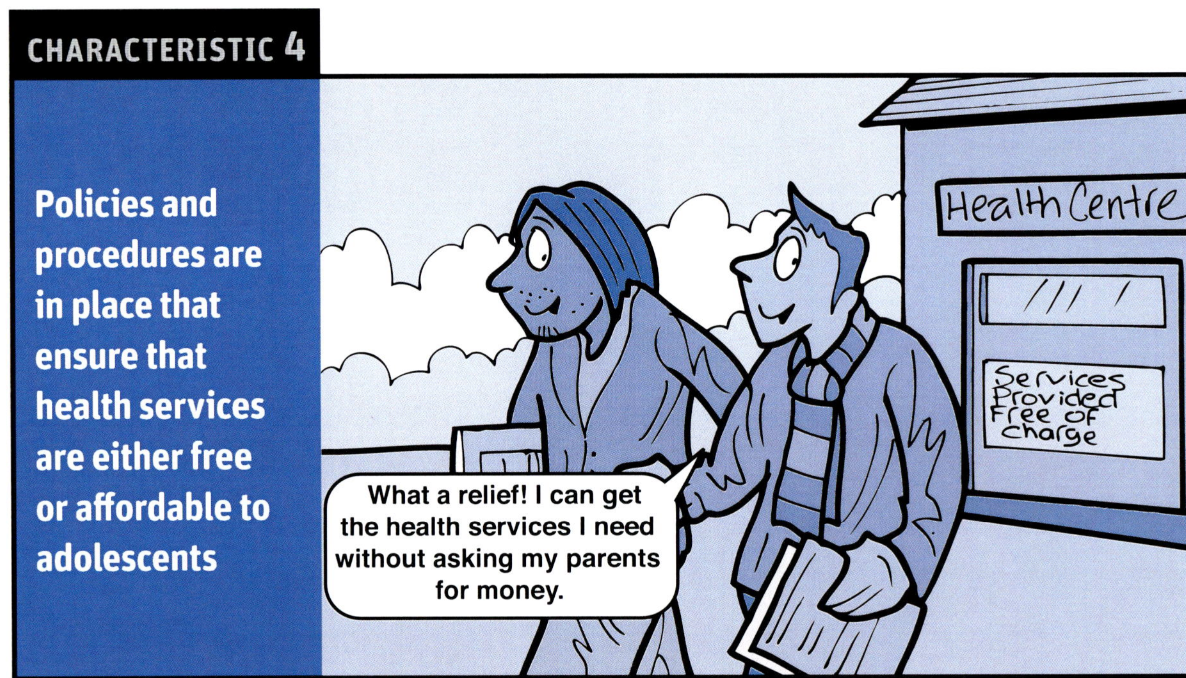

Adolescent client tool:

No.	Question	Response	Score
14	Were you asked to pay for health services?	0=Yes 1=No	Total "No" divided by total number of adolescent clients interviewed
14 a	If you were asked to pay for health services, were you able to pay?	0=No 1=Yes	Total "Yes" divided by total number of adolescent clients interviewed
14 b	In case you could not pay, did you receive the health services anyway?	0=No 1=Yes	Total "Yes" divided by total number of adolescent clients interviewed
	Aggregate adolescent client score		**Total score**

Manager tool:

No.	Question	Response	Score
6	Are fees for adolescent clients less than fees for adult clients?	0=No 1=Yes	Total "Yes" divided by total number of managers interviewed
7	Do you provide concessions for clients who cannot afford to pay for health services?	0=No 1=Yes	Total "Yes" divided by total number of managers interviewed
	Aggregate manager score		**Total score**

Adolescent-in-community tool:

No.	Question	Response	Score
4	Have you or your friends been denied health services at the health facility because you could not pay the fee for the health services?	0=Yes 1=No	Total "No" divided by total number of adolescents in community interviewed
	Aggregate adolescent-in-community score		**Total score**

Overall score on Characteristic 4

	Category	Min – Max	Score
1	**Aggregate adolescent client score**	0 – 3	
2	**Aggregate manager score**	0 – 2	
3	**Aggregate adolescent-in-community score**	0 – 1	
	Absolute total score	0 – 6	
	Relative score for Characteristic 4	0 to 100%	$\left(\frac{\text{Total score}}{6}\right) \times 100$

SCORING SHEETS

CHARACTERISTIC 5
The point of health service delivery has convenient hours of operation
RECEPTION
It's great that you are open during the lunch hour. This makes it very easy for me to come.
TIMINGS

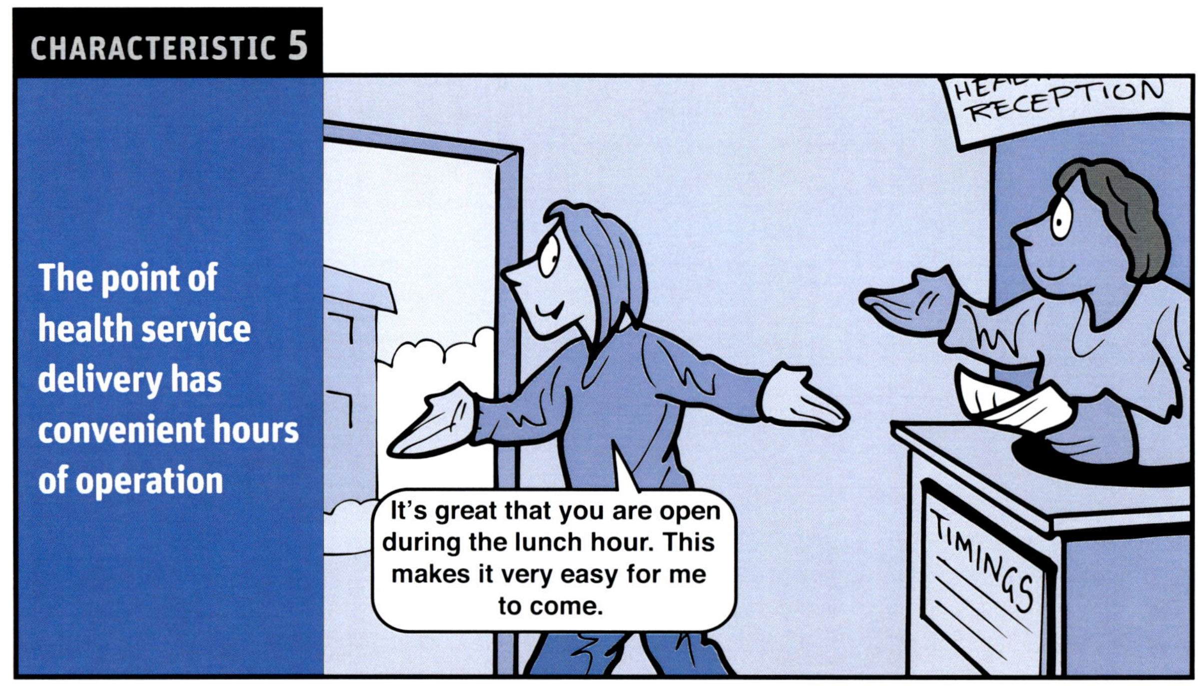

Adolescent client tool:

No.	Question	Response	Score
16	Are the working days and working hours of the health facility convenient for you?	0=No 1=Yes	Total "Yes" divided by total number of adolescent clients interviewed
	Aggregate adolescent client score		**Total score**

Manager tool:

No.	Question	Response	Score
9	Are the working days and working hours of the health facility convenient for adolescents?	0=No 1=Yes	Total "Yes" divided by total number of managers interviewed
	Aggregate manager score		**Total score**

Adolescent-in-community tool:

No.	Question	Response	Score
6	Are the working days and working hours of the health facility convenient for you?	0=Yes 1=No	Total "No" divided by total number of adolescents in community interviewed
	Aggregate adolescent-in-community score		**Total score**

Overall score on Characteristic 5

	Category	Min – Max	Score
1	Aggregate adolescent client score	0 – 1	
2	Aggregate manager score	0 – 1	
3	Aggregate adolescent-in-community score	0 – 1	
	Absolute total score	0 – 3	
	Relative score for Characteristic 5	0 to 100%	$\left(\frac{\text{Total score}}{3}\right) \times 100$

SCORING SHEETS

CHARACTERISTIC 6

Adolescents are well-informed about the range of available reproductive health services and how to obtain them

A nurse talked to us the other day – said we could go to any health centre nearby if we had a problem and wanted information or advice.

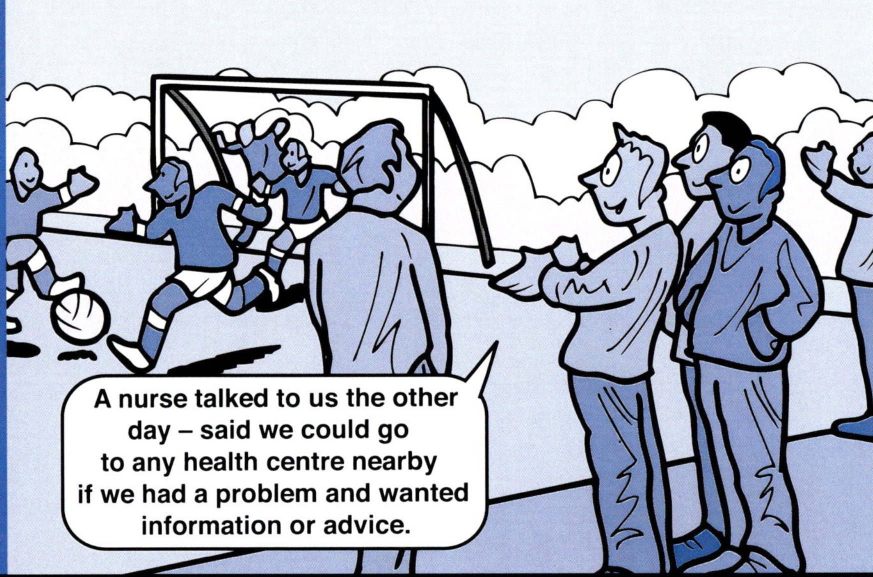

Adolescent client tool:

No.	Question	Response	Score
17	Could you tell me which reproductive health services are offered at this health facility?	0=No 1=Yes	Total "Yes" divided by total number of adolescent clients interviewed
	Aggregate adolescent client score		**Total score**

Adolescent-in-community tool:

No.	Question	Response	Score
8	Could you tell me which reproductive health services are offered at this health facility?	0=No 1=Yes	Total "Yes" divided by total number of adolescents in community interviewed
	Aggregate adolescent-in-community score		**Total score**

Overall score on Characteristic 6

	Category	Min – Max	Score
1	Aggregate adolescent client score	0 – 1	
2	Aggregate adolescent-in-community score	0 – 1	
	Absolute total score	0 – 2	
	Relative score for Characteristic 6	0 to 100%	$\left(\frac{\text{Total score}}{2}\right) \times 100$

SCORING SHEETS

CHARACTERISTIC 7

Community members understand the benefits that adolescents will gain by obtaining the health services they need, and support their provision

So THIS is why the provision of health services can help YOUR adolescents.
HEALTH SERVICE INFO
OK, now I understand. Now I trust and value the provision of health services.

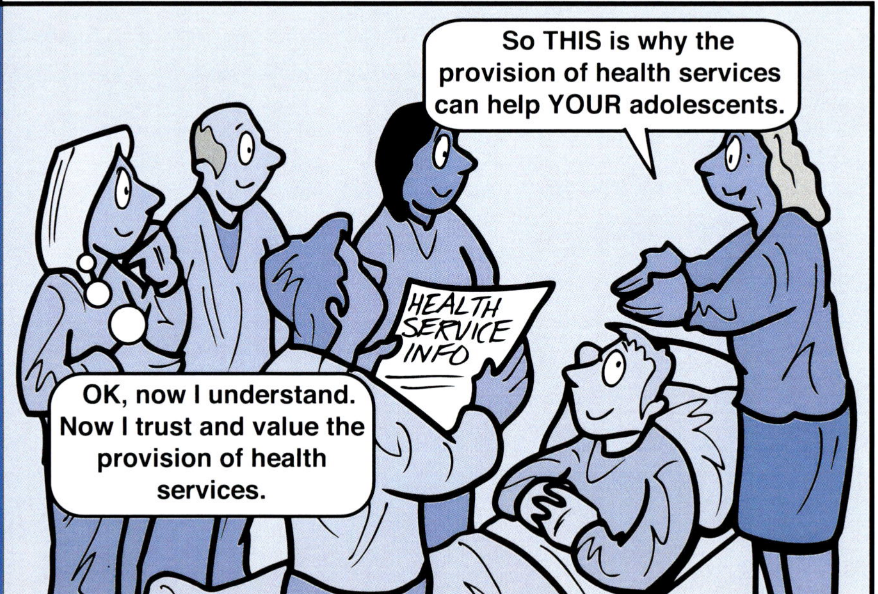

Adolescent client tool:

No.	Question	Response	Score
19	Do you think that your parents/guardians would be supportive of you coming to this health facility for reproductive health services?	0=No 1=Yes	Total "Yes" divided by total number of adolescent clients interviewed
20	Are there some reproductive health services that your parents/ guardians might not want to be provided to you?	0=Yes 1=No	Total "No" divided by total number of adolescent clients interviewed
21	Do you think other adults in the community are supportive of adolescents coming to this health facility for reproductive health services?	0=No 1=Yes	Total "Yes" divided by total number of adolescent clients interviewed
	Aggregate adolescent client score		**Total score**

Health-care provider tool:

No.	Question	Response	Score
8	Do community members support the provision of reproductive health services to adolescents?	0=No 1=Yes	Total "Yes" divided by total number of health-care providers interviewed
	Aggregate health-care provider score		**Total score**

Community member tool:

No.	Question	Response	Score
3	Do you think that adolescents need reproductive health services?	0=No 1=Yes	Total "Yes" divided by total number of community members interviewed
4	Do you believe that adolescents should be provided with reproductive health services?	0=No 1=Yes	Total "Yes" divided by total number of community members interviewed
5	Do you know the reproductive health services that are available to adolescents at this health facility?	0=No 1=Yes	Total "Yes" divided by total number of community members interviewed
6	Are there certain reproductive health services that adolescents should not receive at this health facility?	0=Yes 1=No	Total "No" divided by total number of community members interviewed
	Aggregate community member score		**Total score**

Adolescent-in-community tool:

No.	Question	Response	Score
9	Do you think your parents/guardians would be supportive of you coming to this health facility for reproductive health services?	0=No 1=Yes	Total "Yes" divided by total number of adolescents in community interviewed
10	Are there some reproductive health services that your parents/ guardians might not want to be provided to you?	0=Yes 1=No	Total "No" divided by total number of adolescents in community interviewed
11	Do you think other adults in the community are supportive of adolescents coming to this health facility for reproductive health services?	0=No 1=Yes	Total "Yes" divided by total number of adolescents in community interviewed
	Aggregate adolescent-in-community score		**Total score**

Overall score on Characteristic 7

	Category	Min – Max	Score
1	**Aggregate adolescent client score**	0 – 3	
2	**Aggregate health-care provider score**	0 – 1	
3	**Aggregate community member score**	0 – 4	
4	**Aggregate adolescent-in-community score**	0 – 3	
	Absolute total score	0 – 11	
	Relative score for Characteristic 7	0 to 100%	$\left(\frac{\text{Total score}}{11}\right) \times 100$

SCORING SHEETS

CHARACTERISTIC 8

Some health services and health-related commodities are provided to adolescents in the community by selected community members, outreach workers and adolescents themselves

Restaurant
BAR
DISCO
Protect your self!
It's important that you protect yourselves.

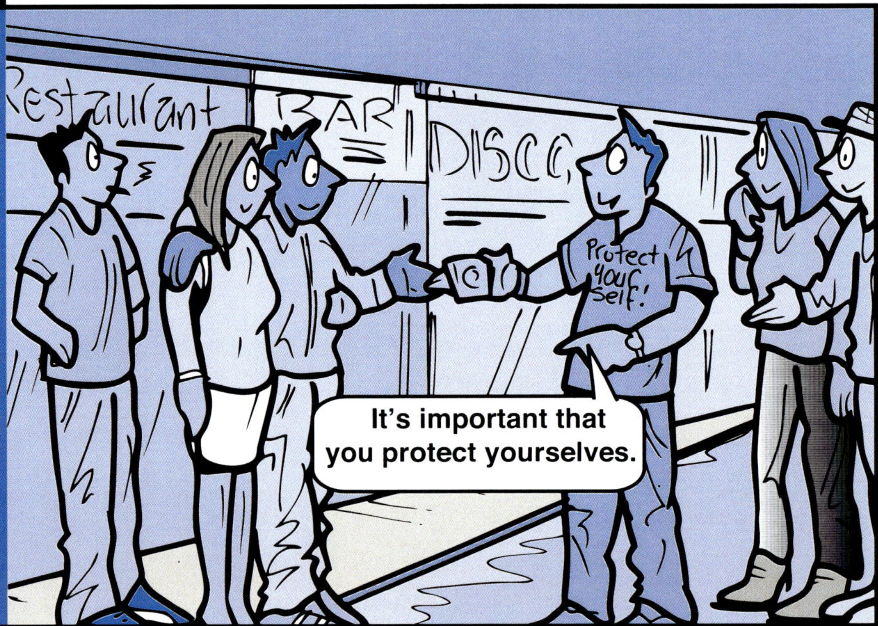

Adolescent client tool:

No.	Question	Response	Score
22	Are you aware of any health services that are provided to adolescents in the community?	0=No 1=Yes	Total "Yes" divided by total number of adolescent clients interviewed
	Aggregate adolescent client score		**Total score**

Manager tool:

No.	Question	Response	Score
10	Do you provide any type of health services to adolescents in the community?	0=No 1=Yes	Total "Yes" divided by the total number of outreach workers interviewed
	Aggregate manager score		**Total score**

Outreach worker tool:

No.	Question	Response	Score
3	Do you provide any type of health services to adolescents in the community?	0=No 1=Yes	Total "Yes" divided by total number of outreach workers interviewed
	Aggregate adolescent client score		**Total score**

Adolescent-in-community tool:

No.	Question	Response	Score
12	Are you aware of any health services that are provided to adolescents in the community?	0=No 1=Yes	Total "Yes" divided by total number of adolescents in community interviewed
13	Are you aware of any adolescents who are involved in providing health services to other adolescents in the community?	0=No 1=Yes	Total "Yes" divided by total number of adolescents in community interviewed
	Aggregate adolescent-in-community score		**Total score**

Overall score on Characteristic 8

	Category	Min – Max	Score
1	**Aggregate adolescent client score**	0 – 1	
2	**Aggregate outreach worker score**	0 – 1	
3	**Aggregate manager score**	0 – 1	
4	**Aggregate adolescent-in-community score**	0 – 2	
	Absolute total score	0 – 5	
	Relative score for Characteristic 8	0 to 100%	$\left(\frac{\text{Total score}}{5}\right) \times 100$

SCORING SHEETS

CHARACTERISTIC 9

Policies and procedures are in place that guarantee client confidentiality

HeathCentre
Confidentiality
Policy
Statement
I don't want anybody to know about my problem.
It's OK, nobody from the health centre will speak loosely about your problem.

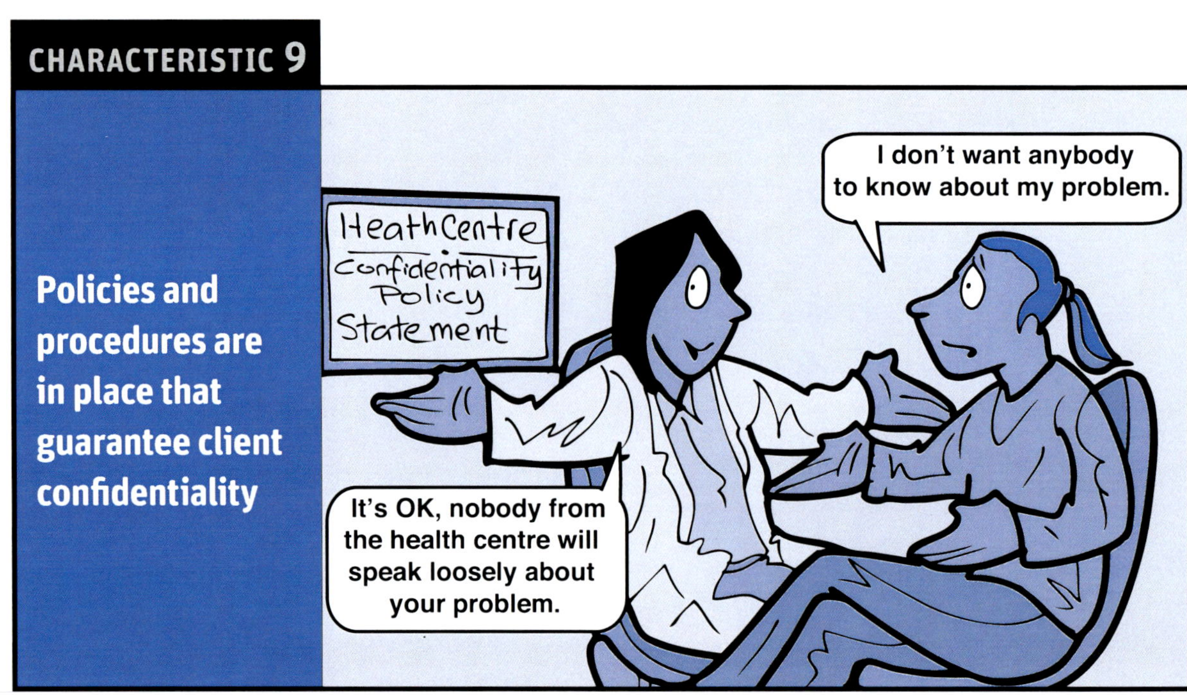

Adolescent client tool:

No.	Question	Response	Score
23	Do you believe that the information you shared with the health-care provider will be kept confidential?	0=No 1=Yes	Total "Yes" divided by total number of adolescent clients interviewed
24	Do you believe that the receptionist or other support staff working there will keep your information confidential?	0=No 1=Yes	Total "Yes" divided by total number of adolescent clients interviewed
25 a	If you tell a doctor something personal, others in the health facility or the community will find out.	0=Yes 1=No	Total "No" divided by total number of adolescent clients interviewed
25 b	If you tell a nurse something personal, others in the health facility or the community will find out.	0=Yes 1=No	Total "No" divided by total number of adolescent clients interviewed
	Aggregate adolescent client score		**Total score**

Health-care provider tool:

No.	Question	Response	Score
9	Are there any policies or procedures in place that guarantee the confidentiality of adolescent clients in this health facility?	0=No 1=Yes	Total "Yes" divided by total number of health-care providers interviewed
	Aggregate health-care provider score		**Total score**

Manager tool:

No.	Question	Response	Score
11	Are there any policies or procedures that guarantee the confidentiality of adolescent clients in this health facility?	0=No 1=Yes	Total "Yes" divided by total number of managers interviewed
	Aggregate manager score		**Total score**

Observation guide:

No.	Question	Response	Score
1	Do written policies and procedures exist for protecting client confidentiality?	0=No 1=Yes	Score 1 for "Yes" or 0 for "No"
	Aggregate observation score		**Total score**

Overall score on Characteristic 9

	Category	Min – Max	Score
1	**Aggregate adolescent client score**	0 – 4	
2	**Aggregate health-care provider score**	0 – 1	
3	**Aggregate manager score**	0 – 1	
4	**Aggregate observation score**	0 – 1	
	Absolute total score	0 – 7	
	Relative score for Characteristic 9	0 to 100%	$\left(\frac{\text{Total score}}{7}\right) \times 100$

SCORING SHEETS

CHARACTERISTIC 10

The point of health service delivery ensures privacy

Health Centre
I feel comfortable coming here. I can come and go without anyone seeing me.
NEWTOWN UNIVERSITY

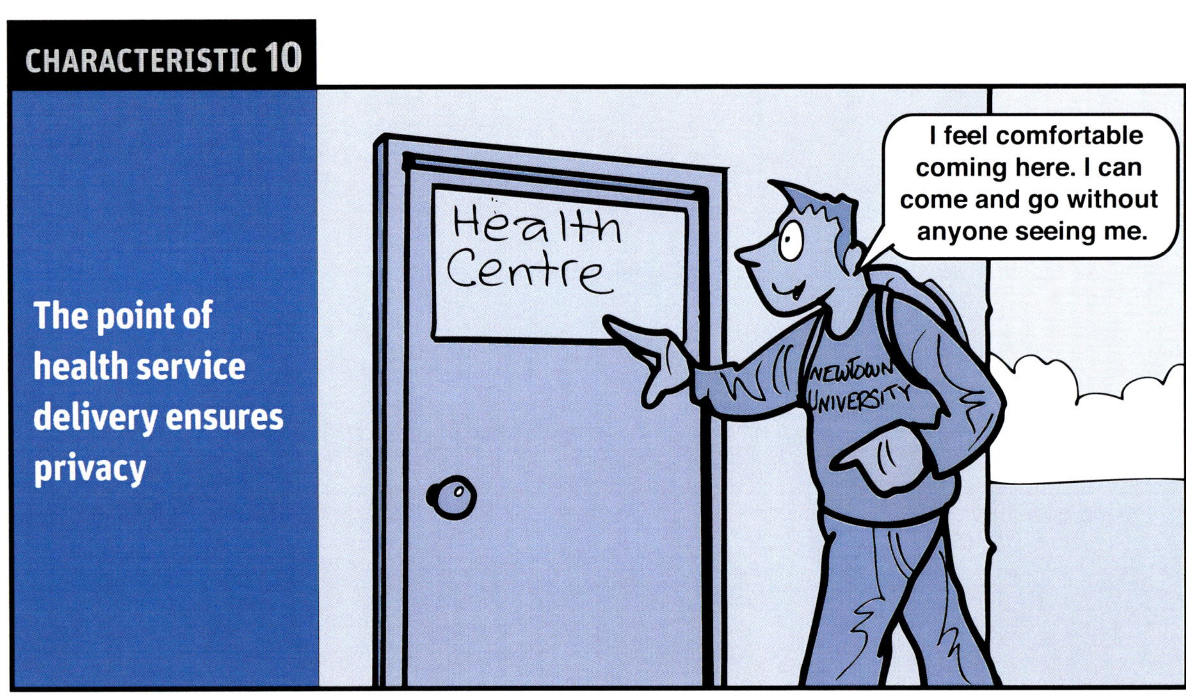

Adolescent client tool:

No.	Question	Response	Score
26	When you visited the health facility, did you believe that other clients could see you and hear you and know what you came for?	0=Yes 1=No	Total "No" divided by total number of adolescent clients interviewed
27	When you were talking to the person at the reception/ registration counter, could other people hear you?	0=Yes 1=No	Total "No" divided by total number of adolescent clients interviewed
28	Did anyone interrupt your discussion with the health-care provider?	0=Yes 1=No	Total "No" divided by total number of adolescent clients interviewed
29	Do you believe that others could hear your discussion with the health-care provider when you were in the consultation/ examination/treatment room?	0=Yes 1=No	Total "No" divided by total number of adolescent clients interviewed
	Aggregate adolescent client score		**Total score**

Health-care provider tool:

No.	Question	Response	Score
11	Are you ever interrupted by other staff when providing services to adolescent clients?	0=Yes 1=No	Total "No" divided by total number of health-care providers interviewed
12	Is it possible for other people to hear your conversations or counselling sessions with adolescent clients?	0=Yes 1=No	Total "No" divided by total number of health-care providers interviewed
	Aggregate health-care provider score		**Total score**

Manager tool:

No.	Question	Response	Score
13	Are there guidelines in place to provide privacy for adolescent clients?	0=No 1=Yes	Total "Yes" divided by total number of managers interviewed
	Aggregate manager score		**Total score**

Observation guide:

No.	Question	Response	Score
3	In the reception area, is it possible to hear the conversations between the receptionist and the adolescent clients?	1=No 0=Yes	Score 1 for "No" or 0 for "Yes"
4	In the waiting area, is it possible to hear the conversations between the receptionist and the adolescent clients?	1=No 0=Yes	Score 1 for "No" or 0 for "Yes"
5	In the consultation/examination/ treatment area, is it possible to hear the conversations between other health-care providers and their adolescent clients?	1=No 0=Yes	Score 1 for "No" or 0 for "Yes"
	Aggregate observation score		**Total score**

Overall score on Characteristic 10

	Category	Min – Max	Score
1	**Aggregate adolescent client score**	0 – 4	
2	**Aggregate health-care provider score**	0 – 2	
3	**Aggregate manager score**	0 – 1	
4	**Aggregate observation score**	0 – 3	
	Absolute total score	0 – 10	
	Relative score for Characteristic 10	0 to 100%	$\left(\frac{\text{Total score}}{10}\right) \times 100$

SCORING SHEETS

CHARACTERISTIC 11

Health-care providers are non-judgmental, considerate, and easy to relate to

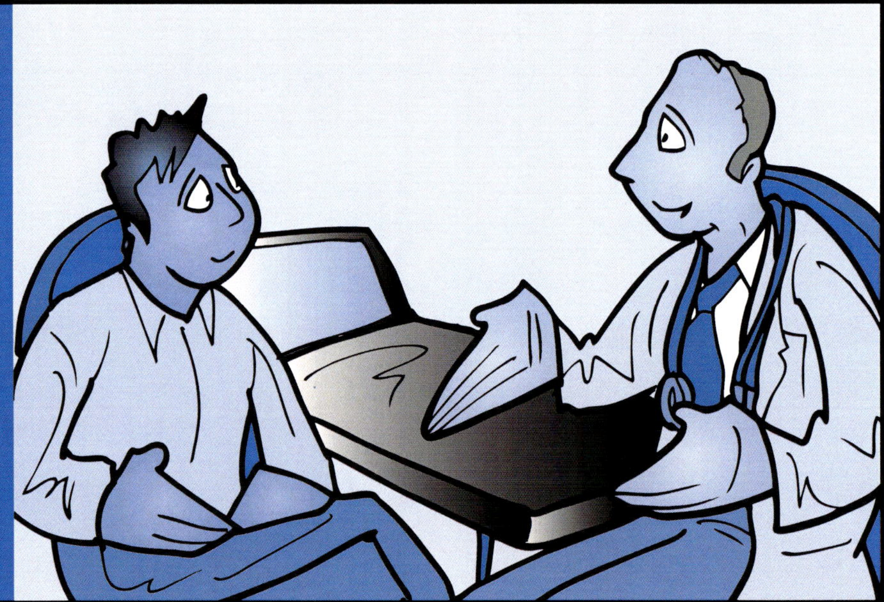

Adolescent client tool:

No.	Question	Response	Score
30	Did the health-care provider give you his/her full attention?	0=No 1=Yes	Total "Yes" divided by total number of adolescent clients interviewed
31	Did the health-care provider seem interested in what you had to say?	0=No 1=Yes	Total "Yes" divided by total number of adolescent clients interviewed
32	Did the health-care provider respect your opinion and decisions even if they were different from his or hers?	0=No 1=Yes	Total "Yes" divided by total number of adolescent clients interviewed
33	Did the health-care provider treat you in a supportive and considerate manner?	0=No 1=Yes	Total "Yes" divided by total number of adolescent clients interviewed
	Aggregate adolescent client score		**Total score**

Observation guide:

No.	Question	Response	Score
7	Did the health-care provider give his/her full attention to the client?	01=No 01=Yes	Score 1 for "No" or 0 for "Yes".
8	Did the health-care provider appear interested in what the client was saying?	01=No 01=Yes	Score 1 for "No" or 0 for "Yes".
9	Did the health-care provider show respect for the opinions of the client?	1=No 0=Yes	Score 1 for "No" or 0 for "Yes"
10	Did the health-care provider treat the client in a supportive and considerate manner?	01=No 01=Yes	Score 1 for "No" or 0 for "Yes".
	Aggregate observation score		**Total score**

Overall score on Characteristic 11

	Category	Min – Max	Score
1	**Aggregate adolescent client score**	0 – 4	
2	**Aggregate observation score**	0 – 4	
	Absolute total score	0 – 10	
	Relative score for Characteristic 11	0 to 100%	$\left(\frac{\text{Total score}}{4}\right) \times 100$

SCORING SHEETS

CHARACTERISTIC 12

The point of health service delivery ensures consultations occur in a short waiting time, with or without an appointment, and (where necessary) swift referral

Adolescent client tool:

No.	Question	Response	Score
34	Have you found the waiting times to see the health-care provider reasonable?	0=No 1=Yes	Total "Yes" divided by total number of adolescent clients interviewed
35a	Did the health-care provider explain to you why you were being referred to another place (if applicable)?	0=No 1=Yes	Total "Yes" divided by total number of adolescent clients interviewed
35b	Did the health-care provider explain to you where and when to go (if applicable)?	0=No 1=Yes	Total "Yes" divided by total number of adolescent clients interviewed
	Aggregate adolescent client score		**Total score**

Health-care provider tool:

No.	Question	Response	Score
13	Do you know the procedures for making referrals for adolescent clients?	0=No 1=Yes	Total "Yes" divided by total number of health-care providers interviewed
14	Are adolescent clients provided with any assistance with the referral?	0=No 1=Yes	Total "Yes" divided by total number of health-care providers interviewed
	Aggregate health-care provider score		**Total score**

Support staff tool:

No.	Question	Response	Score
7	Do you know the procedures for making referrals for adolescent clients?	0=No 1=Yes	Total "Yes" divided by total number of support staff interviewed
8	Are adolescent clients provided with any assistance with the referral?	0=No 1=Yes	Total "Yes" divided by total number of support staff interviewed
	Aggregate support staff score		**Total score**

Observation guide:

No.	Question	Response	Score
12	Did you hear any complaints from adolescent clients about the waiting time?	0=No 1=Yes	Score 1 for "No" and 0 for "Yes"
	Aggregate observation score		**Total score**

Overall score on Characteristic 12

	Category	Min – Max	Score
1	**Aggregate adolescent client score**	0 – 3	
2	**Aggregate health-care provider score**	0 – 2	
3	**Aggregate support staff score**	0 – 2	
4	**Aggregate observation score**	0 – 1	
	Absolute total score	0 – 8	
	Relative score for Characteristic 12	0 to 100%	$\left(\frac{\text{Total score}}{8}\right) \times 100$

SCORING SHEETS

CHARACTERISTIC 13

The point of health service delivery has an appealing and clean environment

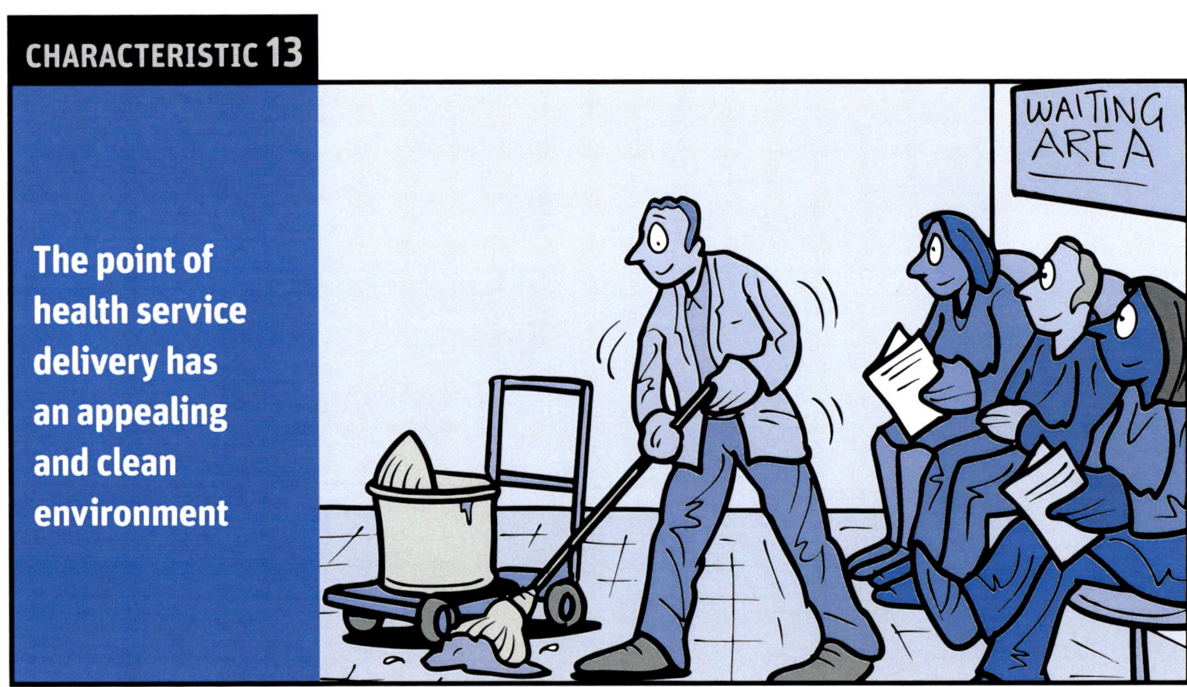

Adolescent client tool:

No.	Question	Response	Score
36	Did you find the health facility a welcoming place to come to?	0= No 1= Yes	Total "Yes" divided by total number of adolescent clients interviewed
37a	Did you find the areas surrounding the health facility to be clean?	0=No 1=Yes	Total "Yes" divided by total number of adolescent clients interviewed
37b	Did you find the reception area of the health facility to be clean?	0=No 1=Yes	Total "Yes" divided by total number of adolescent clients interviewed
37c	Did you find the waiting room of the health facility to be clean?	0=No 1=Yes	Total "Yes" divided by total number of adolescent clients interviewed
37d	Did you find the toilets of the health facility to be clean?	0=No 1=Yes	Total "Yes" divided by total number of adolescent clients interviewed
37e	Did you find the consultation room/examination room of the health facility to be clean?	0=No 1=Yes	Total "Yes" divided by total number of adolescent clients interviewed
	Aggregate adolescent client score		**Total score**

Observation guide:

No.	Question	Response	Score
13a	Are the areas surrounding the health facility clean?	0=No 1=Yes	Score 1 for "Yes" or 0 for "No"
13b	Is the reception area of the health facility clean?	0=No 1=Yes	Score 1 for "Yes" or 0 for "No"
13c	Is the waiting room of the health facility clean?	0=No 1=Yes	Score 1 for "Yes" or 0 for "No"
13d	Are the toilets of the health facility clean?	0=No 1=Yes	Score 1 for "Yes" or 0 for "No"
13e	Is the consultation/examination room of the health facility clean?	0=No 1=Yes	Score 1 for "Yes" or 0 for "No"
14	Does the waiting room have adequate seating for each waiting client?	0=No 1=Yes	Score 1 for "Yes" or 0 for "No"
15	Does the waiting room have lighting sufficient to read?	0=No 1=Yes	Score 1 for "Yes" or 0 for "No"
16	Is the health facility well-ventilated?	0=No 1=Yes	Score 1 for "Yes" or 0 for "No"
17	Is safe drinking-water available for adolescent clients?	0=No 1=Yes	Score 1 for "Yes" or 0 for "No"
	Aggregate observation score		**Total score**

Overall score on Characteristic 13

	Category	Min – Max	Score
1	**Aggregate adolescent client score**	0 – 6	
2	**Aggregate observation score**	0 – 9	
	Absolute total score	0 – 15	
	Relative score for Characteristic 13	0 to 100%	$\left(\frac{\text{Total score}}{15}\right) \times 100$

SCORING SHEETS

CHARACTERISTIC 14

The point of health service delivery provides information and education through a variety of channels

Health Information
Health Info
INF
So THIS is what it's REALLY all about.
This is all so clear and easy to understand.
Please take One!
YOUR health

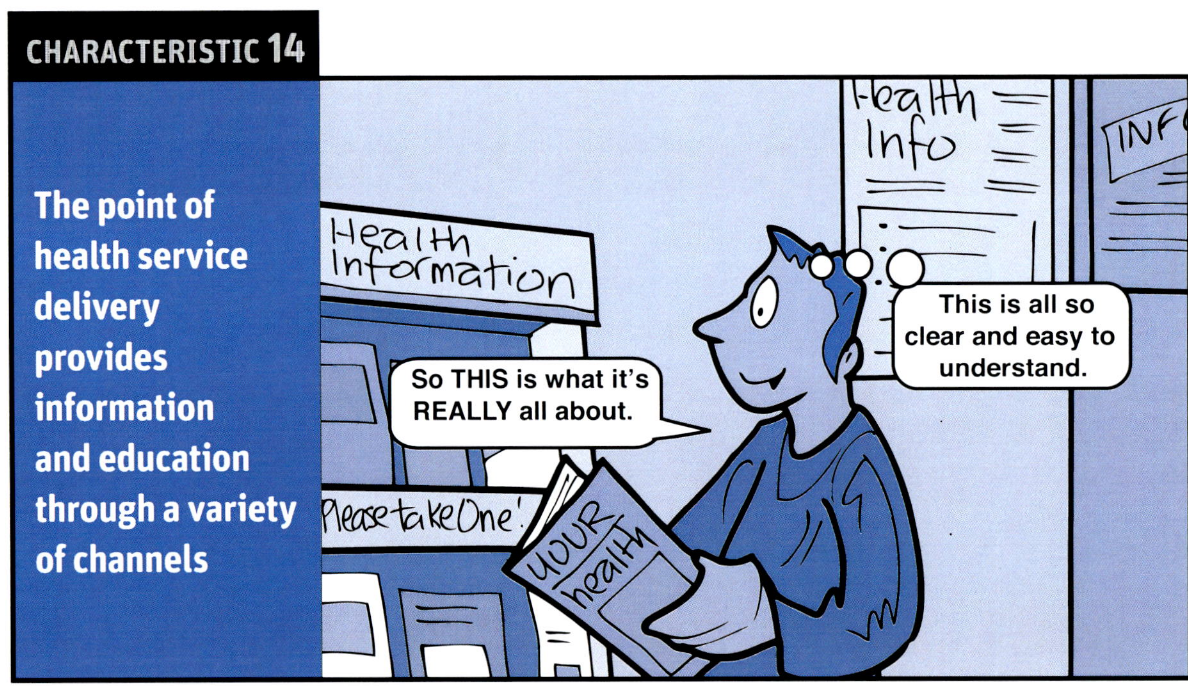

Adolescent client tool:

No.	Question	Response	Score
38	Did you see informational/educational materials on adolescent health topics during your visit to the health facility?	0=No 1=Yes	Total "Yes" divided by total number of adolescent clients interviewed
38a	Did the materials contain information that you found useful?	0=No 1=Yes	Total "Yes" divided by total number of adolescent clients interviewed
38b	Did you find the materials easy to read?	0=No 1=Yes	Total "Yes" divided by total number of adolescent clients interviewed
38c	Did you find the materials interesting to read?	0=No 1=Yes	Total "Yes" divided by total number of adolescent clients interviewed
	Aggregate adolescent client score		**Total score**

Manager tool:

No.	Question	Response	Score
14	Are there informational and educational materials available for adolescents in the waiting room?	0=No 1=Yes	Total "Yes" divided by total number of managers interviewed
	Aggregate manager score		**Total score**

Observation guide:

No.	Question	Response	Score
18	Are there any informational and educational materials that adolescents can read/watch while they are waiting?	0=No 1=Yes	Score 1 for "Yes" or 0 for "No"
19	Are there any signs or posters in the health facility that target adolescents?	0=No 1=Yes	Score 1 for "Yes" and 0 for "No"
	Aggregate observation score		**Total score**

Overall score on Characteristic 14

	Category	Min – Max	Score
1	**Aggregate adolescent client score**	0 – 4	
2	**Aggregate manager score**	0 – 1	
3	**Aggregate observation score**	0 – 2	
	Absolute total score	0 – 7	
	Relative score for Characteristic 14	0 to 100%	$\left(\frac{\text{Total score}}{7}\right) \times 100$

SCORING SHEETS

CHARACTERISTIC 15

Adolescents are actively involved in designing, assessing and providing health services

Health Centre Waiting Room
The last time I gave them a suggestion, they acted on it.
MY Suggestion
Place your suggestions here
FEED BACK BOX

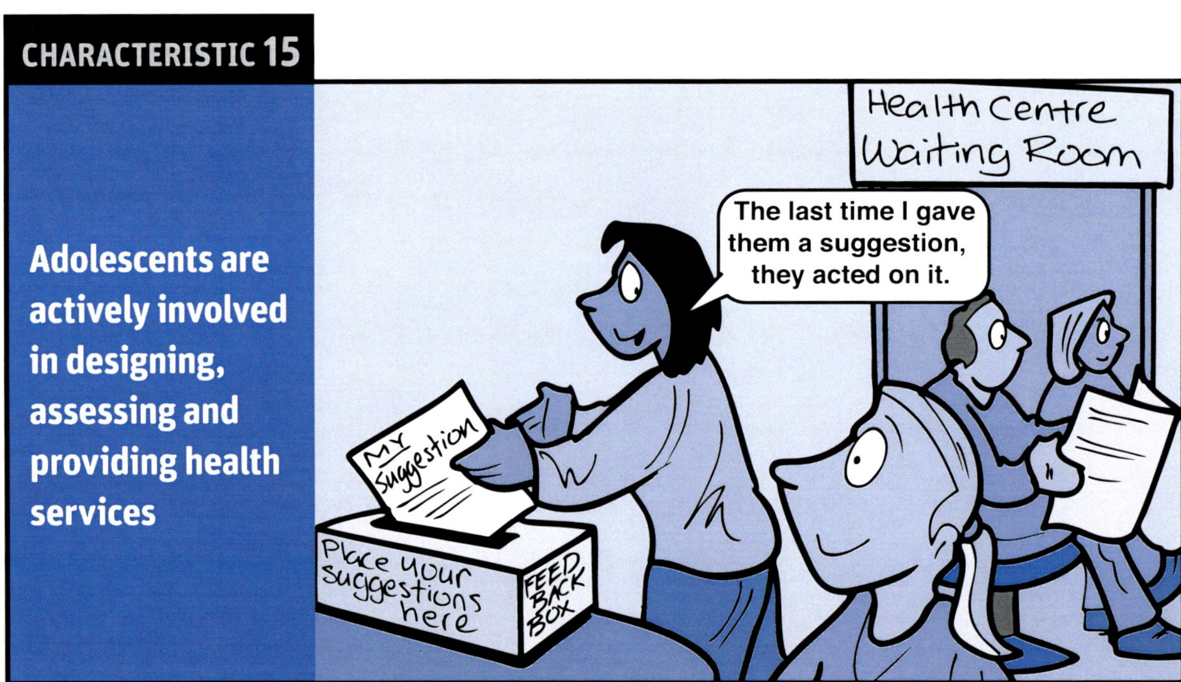

Adolescent client tool:

No.	Question	Response	Score
39	Are you aware of adolescents who were/are involved in contributing to decisions about how health services should be delivered to adolescent clients?	0=No 1=Yes	Total "Yes" divided by total number of adolescent clients interviewed
40	Do you believe that you could make a suggestion to the staff for improving the way in which health services are delivered here?	0=No 1=Yes	Total "Yes" divided by total number of adolescent clients interviewed
	Aggregate adolescent client score		**Total score**

Manager tool:

No.	Question	Response	Score
15	Do you give adolescents opportunities to suggest/recommend changes to make services more responsive to adolescent clients?	0=No 1=Yes	Total "Yes" divided by total number of managers interviewed
16	In addition to being consulted as clients, are adolescents currently involved in decision-making about how health services are delivered to adolescents?	0=No 1=Yes	Total "Yes" divided by total number of managers interviewed
	Aggregate manager score		**Total score**

Overall score on Characteristic 15

	Category	Min – Max	Score
1	**Aggregate adolescent client score**	0 – 2	
2	**Aggregate manager score**	0 – 2	
	Absolute total score	0 – 4	
	Relative score for Characteristic 15	0 to 100%	$\left(\frac{\text{Total score}}{4}\right) \times 100$

CHARACTERISTIC 16

The required package of health care is provided to fulfil the needs of all adolescents either at the point of health service delivery or through referral linkages

Health Centre
We deal with the issues our adolescents come to us with ourselves. We also have good links with the local hospital and can send patients for treatment there if we can't provide it here.

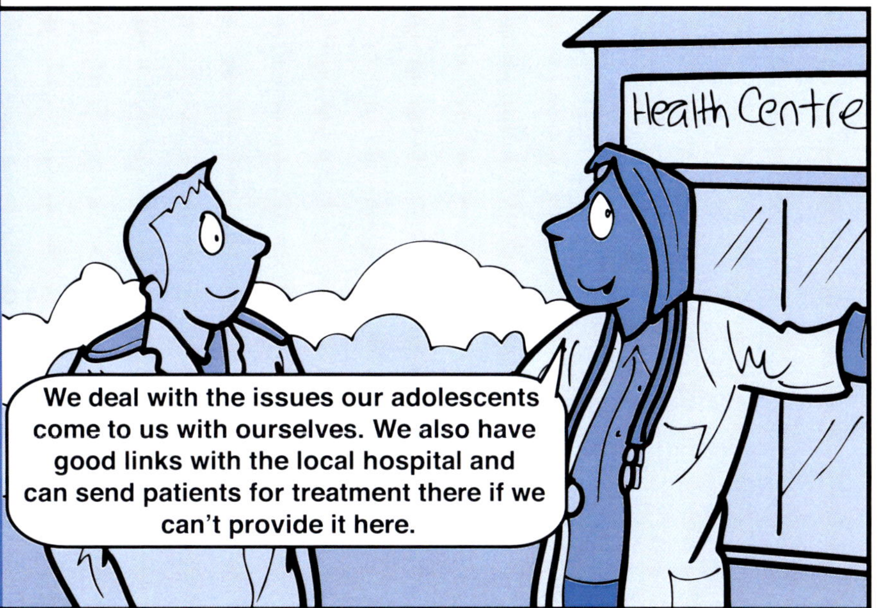

SCORING SHEETS

Adolescent client tool:

No.	Question	Response	Score
41	Did you receive the health service you need to deal with your health concern or health problem?	0=No 1=Yes	Total "Yes" divided by total number of adolescent clients interviewed
42	Were you referred to another health facility for health services not available at this one?	0=No 1=Yes	Total "Yes" divided by total number of adolescent clients interviewed
	Aggregate adolescent client score		**Total score**

Health-care provider tool:

No.	Question	Response	Score
15a	Are adolescent clients offered information and counselling on reproductive health, sexuality and safe sex?	0=No 1=Yes	Total "Yes" divided by total number of health-care providers interviewed
15b	Are adolescent clients offered testing and counselling services for HIV?	0=No 1=Yes	Total "Yes" divided by total number of health-care providers interviewed
15c	Are adolescent clients offered STI/RTI diagnostic services, including laboratory tests where available?	0=No 1=Yes	Total "Yes" divided by total number of health-care providers interviewed
15d	Are adolescent clients offered pregnancy diagnostic services, including laboratory tests where available?	0=No 1=Yes	Total "Yes" divided by total number of health-care providers interviewed

Continues...

Continued from previous page

No.	Question	Response	Score
15e	Are adolescent clients offered treatment services for STIs/RTIs?	0=No 1=Yes	Total "Yes" divided by total number of health-care providers interviewed
15f	Are adolescent clients offered care during pregnancy?	0=No 1=Yes	Total "Yes" divided by total number of health-care providers interviewed
15g	Are adolescent clients offered care during childbirth?	0=No 1=Yes	Total "Yes" divided by total number of health-care providers interviewed
15h	Are adolescent clients offered care after childbirth?	0=No 1=Yes	Total "Yes" divided by total number of health-care providers interviewed
15i	Are adolescent clients offered abortion services (where they are legal)?	0=No 1=Yes	Total "Yes" divided by total number of health-care providers interviewed
15j	Are adolescent clients offered information and counselling on contraception, including emergency contraception?	0=No 1=Yes	Total "Yes" divided by total number of health-care providers interviewed
15k	Is information and counselling provided on condoms to adolescent clients?	0=No 1=Yes	Total "Yes" divided by total number of health-care providers interviewed
15l	Are HIV-positive adolescents offered care and support services?	0=No 1=Yes	Total "Yes" divided by total number of health-care providers interviewed
15m	Are adolescent clients who have been physically or sexually assaulted offered care and support services?	0=No 1=Yes	Total "Yes" divided by total number of health-care providers interviewed
16	If some services are not available at your health facility, do you know how and where to refer clients for these services?	0=No 1=Yes	Total "Yes" divided by total number of health-care providers interviewed
	Aggregate health-care provider score		**Total score**

RTI = respiratory tract infection; STI = sexually transmitted infection.

Manager tool:

No.	Question	Response	Score
17a	Are adolescent clients offered information and counselling on reproductive health, sexuality and safe sex?	0=No 1=Yes	Score 1 for "Yes" or 0 for "No"
17b	Are adolescent clients offered counselling and testing services for HIV?	0=No 1=Yes	Score 1 for "Yes" or 0 for "No"
17c	Are adolescent clients offered STI/RTI diagnostic services, including laboratory tests where available?	0=No 1=Yes	Score 1 for "Yes" or 0 for "No"
17d	Are adolescent clients offered pregnancy diagnostic services, including laboratory tests were available?	0=No 1=Yes	Score 1 for "Yes" or 0 for "No"
17e	Are adolescent clients offered treatment services for STIs/RTIs?	0=No 1=Yes	Score 1 for "Yes" or 0 for "No"
17f	Are adolescent clients offered care during pregnancy?	0=No 1=Yes	Score 1 for "Yes" or 0 for "No"
17g	Are adolescent clients offered care during childbirth?	0=No 1=Yes	Score 1 for "Yes" or 0 for "No"
17h	Are adolescent clients offered care after childbirth?	0=No 1=Yes	Score 1 for "Yes" or 0 for "No"
17i	Are adolescent clients offered abortion services (where they are legal)?	0=No 1=Yes	Score 1 for "Yes" or 0 for "No"
17j	Are adolescent clients offered information and counselling on contraception, including emergency contraception?	0=No 1=Yes	Score 1 for "Yes" or 0 for "No"
17k	Is information and counselling on condoms provided to adolescent clients?	0=No 1=Yes	Score 1 for "Yes" or 0 for "No"
17l	Are HIV-positive adolescents offered care and support services?	0=No 1=Yes	Score 1 for "Yes" or 0 for "No"
17m	Are adolescent clients who have been physically or sexually assaulted offered care and support services?	0=No 1=Yes	Score 1 for "Yes" or 0 for "No"
18	If some services are not available, do your staff know how and where to refer clients for these services?	0=No 1=Yes	Score 1 for "Yes" or 0 for "No"
	Aggregate health-care provider score		**Total score**

Overall score on Characteristic 16

	Category	Min – Max	Score
1	**Aggregate adolescent client score**	0 – 2	
2	**Aggregate health-care provider score**	0 – 14	
3	**Aggregate manager score**	0 – 14	
	Absolute total score	0 – 30	
	Relative score for Characteristic 16	0 to 100%	$\left(\frac{\text{Total score}}{30}\right) \times 100$

SCORING SHEETS

CHARACTERISTIC 17

Health-care providers have the required competencies to work with adolescents and to provide them with the required health services

Health Centre Consultation Room
Trained in Adolescent Health Care
Thank you very much for explaining everything so clearly.

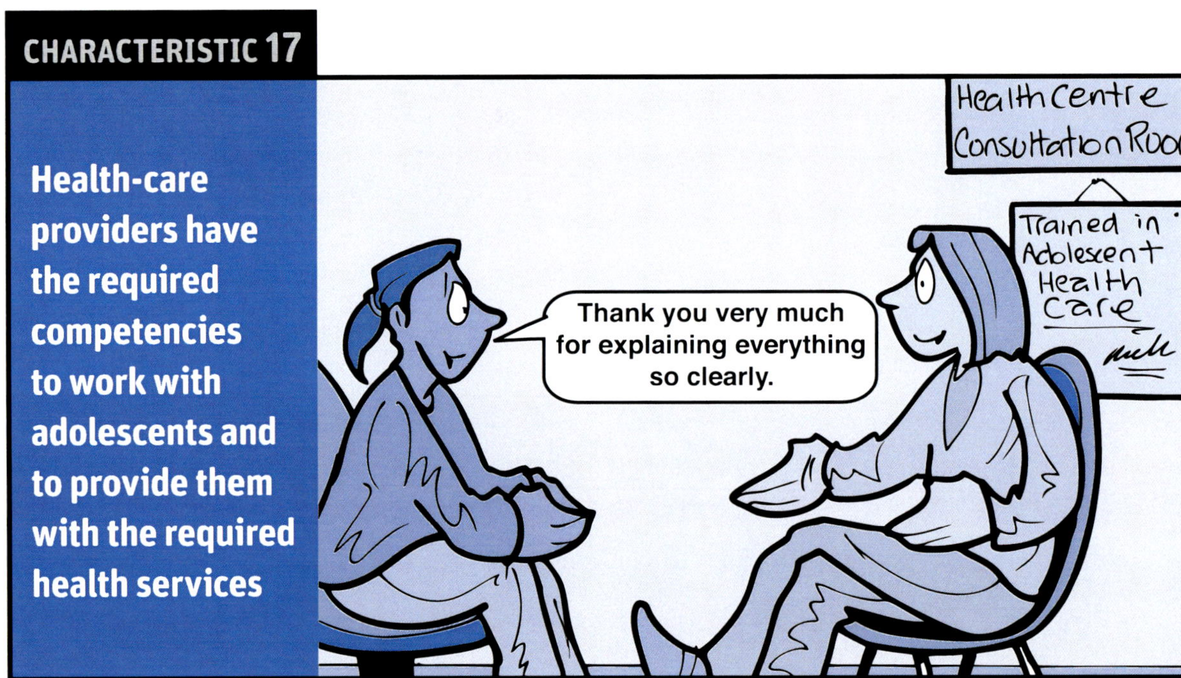

Adolescent client tool:

No.	Question	Response	Score
43	Did the health-care provider explain things in a way you could understand?	0=No 1=Yes	Total "Yes" divided by total number of adolescent clients interviewed
44a	Did the health-care provider explain what check-ups/tests he or she was doing?	0=No 1=Yes	Total "Yes" divided by total number of adolescent clients interviewed
44b	Did the health-care provider explain the results of the check-ups/tests?	0=No 1=Yes	Total "Yes" divided by total number of adolescent clients interviewed
44c	Did the health-care provider explain what treatment he or she was proposing and why (if applicable)?	0=No 1=Yes	Total "Yes" divided by total number of adolescent clients interviewed
45a	Did the health-care provider discuss the pros and cons of the different treatment approaches with you (if applicable)?	0=No 1=Yes	Total "Yes" divided by total number of adolescent clients interviewed
45b	Did the health-care provider ask you what treatment option you preferred (if applicable)?	0=No 1=Yes	Total "Yes" divided by total number of adolescent clients interviewed
	Aggregate adolescent client score		**Total score**

Health-care provider tool:

No.	Question	Response	Score
17a	Do you believe that you have adequate knowledge and skills to provide information and counselling on reproductive health, sexuality and safe sex to adolescent clients?	0=No 1=Yes	Total "Yes" divided by total number of health-care providers interviewed
17b	Do you believe that you have adequate knowledge and skills to provide counselling and testing services for HIV to adolescent clients?	0=No 1=Yes	Total "Yes" divided by total number of health-care providers interviewed
17c	Do you believe that you have adequate knowledge and skills to diagnose adolescent clients for STIs/RTIs, including carrying out laboratory tests where available?	0=No 1=Yes	Total "Yes" divided by total number of health-care providers interviewed
17d	Do you believe that you have adequate knowledge and skills to diagnose pregnancy in your adolescent clients, including carrying out laboratory tests where available?	0=No 1=Yes	Total "Yes" divided by total number of health-care providers interviewed
17e	Do you believe that you have adequate knowledge and skills to treat STIs/RTIs among adolescent clients?	0=No 1=Yes	Total "Yes" divided by total number of health-care providers interviewed
17f	Do you believe that you have adequate knowledge and skills to provide care to adolescent clients during their pregnancy?	0=No 1=Yes	Total "Yes" divided by total number of health-care providers interviewed
17g	Do you believe that you have adequate knowledge and skills to provide care to adolescent clients during their childbirth?	0=No 1=Yes	Total "Yes" divided by total number of health-care providers interviewed
17h	Do you believe that you have adequate knowledge and skills to provide care to adolescent clients after their childbirth?	0=No 1=Yes	Total "Yes" divided by total number of health-care providers interviewed
17i	Do you believe that you have adequate knowledge and skills to provide abortion services to adolescent clients (where they are legal)?	0=No 1=Yes	Total "Yes" divided by total number of health-care providers interviewed
17j	Do you believe that you have adequate knowledge and skills to provide information and counselling on contraception, including emergency contraception, to adolescent clients?	0=No 1=Yes	Total "Yes" divided by total number of health-care providers interviewed
17k	Do you believe that you have adequate knowledge and skills to provide information and counselling on condoms to adolescent clients?	0=No 1=Yes	Total "Yes" divided by total number of health-care providers interviewed
17l	Do you believe that you have adequate knowledge and skills to provide care and support to HIV-positive adolescents?	0=No 1=Yes	Total "Yes" divided by total number of health-care providers interviewed
17m	Do you believe that you have adequate knowledge and skills to provide care and support to adolescent clients who have been physically or sexually assaulted?	0=No 1=Yes	Total "Yes" divided by total number of health-care providers interviewed

Continues...

Continued from previous page

No.	Question	Response	Score
18	Do you believe that you are able/trained to communicate with adolescents about the risks, benefits and potential complications of the treatments and procedures you provide?	0=No 1=Yes	Total "Yes" divided by total number of health-care providers interviewed
19	Do you tell adolescent clients about alternatives to such procedures/treatments?	0=No 1=Yes	Total "Yes" divided by total number of health-care providers interviewed
	Aggregate health-care provider score		**Total score**

Manager tool:

No.	Question	Response	Score
19a	Do your staff have the knowledge and skills to provide information and counselling on reproductive health, sexuality and safe sex to adolescent clients?	0=No 1=Yes	Score 1 for "Yes" or 0 for "No"
19b	Do your staff have the knowledge and skills to provide counselling and testing for HIV to adolescent clients?	0=No 1=Yes	Score 1 for "Yes" or 0 for "No"
19c	Do your staff have the knowledge and skills to diagnose STIs/ RTIs in adolescent clients, and to carry out laboratory tests where available?	0=No 1=Yes	Score 1 for "Yes" or 0 for "No"
19d	Do your staff have the knowledge and skills to diagnose pregnancy in adolescent clients, and to carry out laboratory tests where available?	0=No 1=Yes	Score 1 for "Yes" or 0 for "No"
19e	Do your staff have the knowledge and skills to provide treatment of STIs and RTIs to adolescent clients?	0=No 1=Yes	Score 1 for "Yes" or 0 for "No"
19f	Do your staff have the knowledge and skills to provide care during pregnancy to adolescent clients?	0=No 1=Yes	Score 1 for "Yes" or 0 for "No"
19g	Do your staff have the knowledge and skills to provide care during childbirth to adolescent clients?	0=No 1=Yes	Score 1 for "Yes" or 0 for "No"
19h	Do your staff have the knowledge and skills to provide care after childbirth to adolescent clients?	0=No 1=Yes	Score 1 for "Yes" or 0 for "No"
19i	Do your staff have the knowledge and skills to provide abortion services to adolescent clients (where they are legal)?	0=No 1=Yes	Score 1 for "Yes" or 0 for "No"
19j	Do your staff have the knowledge and skills to provide information and counselling on contraception, including emergency contraception to adolescent clients?	0=No 1=Yes	Score 1 for "Yes" or 0 for "No"
19k	Do your staff have the knowledge and skills to provide information and counselling on condoms to adolescent clients?	0=No 1=Yes	Score 1 for "Yes" or 0 for "No"
19l	Do your staff have the knowledge and skills to provide care and support for HIV-positive adolescents?	0=No 1=Yes	Score 1 for "Yes" or 0 for "No"
19m	Do your staff have the knowledge and skills to provide care and support for adolescent clients who have been physically or sexually assaulted?	0=No 1=Yes	Score 1 for "Yes" or 0 for "No"
	Aggregate manager score		**Total score**

Observation guide:

No.	Question	Response	Score
20a	Did the health-care provider have adequate knowledge and skills to provide information and counselling on reproductive health, sexuality and safe sex to adolescent clients (if applicable)?	0=No 1=Yes	Score 1 for "Yes" or 0 for "No"
20b	Did the health-care provider have adequate knowledge and skills to provide counselling and testing for HIV to adolescent clients (if applicable)?	0=No 1=Yes	Score 1 for "Yes" or 0 for "No"
20c	Did the health-care provider have adequate knowledge and skills to diagnose STIs/RTIs in adolescent clients and to carry out laboratory tests if available (if applicable)?	0=No 1=Yes	Score 1 for "Yes" or 0 for "No"
20d	Did the health-care provider have adequate knowledge and skills to diagnose pregnancy in adolescent clients and to carry out laboratory tests if available (if applicable)?	0=No 1=Yes	Score 1 for "Yes" or 0 for "No"
20e	Did the health-care provider have adequate knowledge and skills to provide treatment of STIs/RTIs to adolescent clients (if applicable)?	0=No 1=Yes	Score 1 for "Yes" or 0 for "No"
20f	Did the health-care provider have adequate knowledge and skills to provide care to adolescent clients during their pregnancy (if applicable)?	0=No 1=Yes	Score 1 for "Yes" or 0 for "No"
20g	Did the health-care provider have adequate knowledge and skills to provide care to adolescent clients during their childbirth (if applicable)?	0=No 1=Yes	Score 1 for "Yes" or 0 for "No"
20h	Did the health-care provider have adequate knowledge and skills to provide care to adolescent clients after their childbirth (if applicable)?	0=No 1=Yes	Score 1 for "Yes" or 0 for "No"
20i	Did the health-care provider have adequate knowledge and skills to provide abortion services to adolescent clients (where they are legal) (if applicable)?	0=No 1=Yes	Score 1 for "Yes" or 0 for "No"
20j	Did the health-care provider have adequate knowledge and skills to provide information and counselling about contraception, including emergency contraception to adolescent clients (if applicable)?	0=No 1=Yes	Score 1 for "Yes" or 0 for "No"
20k	Did the health-care provider have adequate knowledge and skills to provide information and counselling on condoms to adolescent clients (if applicable)?	0=No 1=Yes	Score 1 for "Yes" or 0 for "No"
20l	Did the health-care provider have adequate knowledge and skills to provide care and support for HIV-positive adolescents (if applicable)?	0=No 1=Yes	Score 1 for "Yes" or 0 for "No"
20m	Did the health-care provider have adequate knowledge and skills to provide care and support for adolescents who have been physically or sexually assaulted (if applicable)?	0=No 1=Yes	Score 1 for "Yes" or 0 for "No"
21a	Did the health-care provider communicate with the adolescent client about what check-ups/tests he or she was doing?	0=No 1=Yes	Score 1 for "Yes" or 0 for "No"
21b	Did the health-care provider communicate with the adolescent client about the results of the check-ups/tests?	0=No	Score 1 for "Yes" or 0 for "No"
21c	Did the health-care provider communicate with the adolescent client about treatment he or she was proposing and why (if applicable)?	0=No 1=Yes	Score 1 for "Yes" or 0 for "No"
22	Did the health-care provider tell the adolescent client about alternatives to such procedures and treatments (if applicable)?	0=No 1=Yes	Score 1 for "Yes" or 0 for "No"
	Aggregate observation score		**Total score**

Overall score on Characteristic 17

	Category	Min – Max	Score
1	Aggregate adolescent client score	0 – 6	
2	Aggregate health-care provider score	0 – 15	
3	Aggregate manager score	0 – 13	
4	Aggregate observation score	0 – 17	
	Absolute total score	0 – 51	
	Relative score for Characteristic 17	0 to 100%	$\left(\frac{\text{Total score}}{53}\right) \times 100$

CHARACTERISTIC 18

Health-care providers use evidence-based protocols and guidelines to provide health services

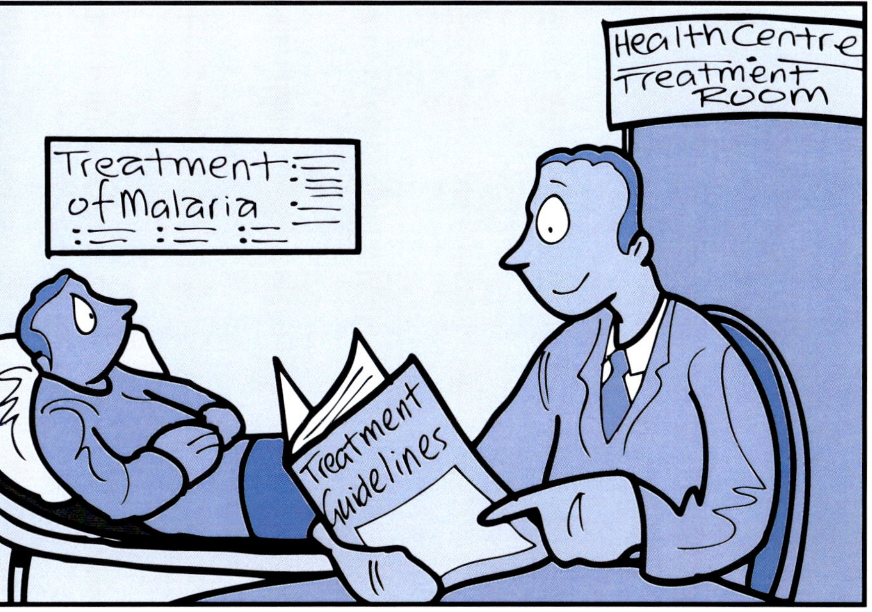

Health-care provider tool:

No.	Question	Response	Score
20a	Do you use protocols and guidelines at your health facility for information and counselling on reproductive health, sexuality and safe sex for adolescent clients?	0=No 1=Yes	Total "Yes" divided by total number of health-care providers interviewed
20b	Do you use protocols and guidelines at your health facility for providing counselling and testing for HIV to adolescent clients?	0=No 1=Yes	Total "Yes" divided by total number of health-care providers interviewed
20c	Do you use protocols and guidelines at your health facility for diagnosing STIs/RTIs in adolescent clients?	0=No 1=Yes	Total "Yes" divided by total number of health-care providers interviewed
20d	Do you use protocols and guidelines at your health facility for diagnosing pregnancy in adolescent clients?	0=No 1=Yes	Total "Yes" divided by total number of health-care providers interviewed
20e	Do you use protocols and guidelines at your health facility for treating STIs/RTIs among adolescent clients?	0=No 1=Yes	Total "Yes" divided by total number of health-care providers interviewed
20f	Do you use protocols and guidelines at your health facility for providing care to adolescent clients during their pregnancy?	0=No 1=Yes	Total "Yes" divided by total number of health-care providers interviewed
20g	Do you use protocols and guidelines at your health facility for providing care to adolescent clients during their childbirth?	0=No 1=Yes	Total "Yes" divided by total number of health-care providers interviewed
20h	Do you use protocols and guidelines at your health facility for providing care to adolescent clients after their childbirth?	0=No 1=Yes	Total "Yes" divided by total number of health-care providers interviewed

Continues...

Continued from previous page

No.	Question	Response	Score
20i	Do you use protocols and guidelines at your health facility for providing abortion services to adolescent clients (where they are legal)?	0=No 1=Yes	Total "Yes" divided by total number of health-care providers interviewed
20j	Do you use protocols and guidelines at your health facility for information and counselling on contraception, including emergency contraception, to adolescent clients?	0=No 1=Yes	Total "Yes" divided by total number of health-care providers interviewed
20k	Do you use protocols and guidelines at your health facility for information and counselling on condoms to adolescent clients?	0=No 1=Yes	Total "Yes" divided by total number of health-care providers interviewed
20l	Do you use protocols and guidelines at your health facility for care and support of HIV-positive adolescents?	0=No 1=Yes	Total "Yes" divided by total number of health-care providers interviewed
20m	Do you use protocols and guidelines at your health facility for care and support of adolescent clients who have been physically or sexually assaulted?	0=No 1=Yes	Total "Yes" divided by total number of health-care providers interviewed
	Aggregate health-care provider score		**Total score**

Manager tool:

No.	Question	Response	Score
20a	Do you use protocols and guidelines at your health facility for information and counselling on reproductive health, sexuality and safe sex for adolescent clients?	0=No 1=Yes	Score 1 for "Yes" or 0 for "No"
20b	Do you use protocols and guidelines at your health facility for counselling and testing for HIV to adolescent clients?	0=No 1=Yes	Score 1 for "Yes" or 0 for "No"
20c	Do you use protocols and guidelines at your health facility for diagnosing STIs/RTIs in adolescent clients?	0=No 1=Yes	Score 1 for "Yes" or 0 for "No"
20d	Do you use protocols and guidelines at your health facility for diagnosing pregnancy in adolescent clients?	0=No 1=Yes	Score 1 for "Yes" or 0 for "No"
20e	Do you use protocols and guidelines at your health facility for treating STIs/RTIs among adolescent clients?	0=No 1=Yes	Score 1 for "Yes" or 0 for "No"
20f	Do you use protocols and guidelines at your health facility for providing care to adolescent clients during their pregnancy?	0=No 1=Yes	Score 1 for "Yes" or 0 for "No"
20g	Do you use protocols and guidelines at your health facility for providing care to adolescent clients during their childbirth?	0=No 1=Yes	Score 1 for "Yes" or 0 for "No"
20h	Do you use protocols and guidelines at your health facility for providing care to adolescent clients after their childbirth?	0=No 1=Yes	Score 1 for "Yes" or 0 for "No"

Continues...

Continued from previous page

No.	Question	Response	Score
20i	Do you use protocols and guidelines at your health facility for providing abortion services to adolescent clients (where they are legal)?	0=No 1=Yes	Score 1 for "Yes" or 0 for "No"
20j	Do you use protocols and guidelines at your health facility for providing information and counselling on contraception, including emergency contraception, to adolescent clients?	0=No 1=Yes	Score 1 for "Yes" or 0 for "No"
20k	Do you use protocols and guidelines at your health facility for providing information and counselling on condoms to adolescent clients?	0=No 1=Yes	Score 1 for "Yes" or 0 for "No"
20l	Do you use protocols and guidelines at your health facility for care and support to HIV-positive adolescents?	0=No 1=Yes	Score 1 for "Yes" or 0 for "No"
20m	Do you use protocols and guidelines at your health facility for care and support of adolescent clients who have been physically or sexually assaulted?	0=No 1=Yes	Score 1 for "Yes" or 0 for "No"
	Aggregate manager score		**Total score**

Observation guide:

No.	Question	Response	Score
23a	Are there protocols and guidelines for information and counselling on reproductive health, sexuality and safe sex to adolescent clients?	0=No 1=Yes	Score 1 for "Yes" or 0 for "No"
23b	Are there protocols and guidelines for providing counselling and testing services for HIV to adolescent clients?	0=No 1=Yes	Score 1 for "Yes" or 0 for "No"
23c	Are there protocols and guidelines for diagnosing STIs/RTIs in adolescent clients?	0=No 1=Yes	Score 1 for "Yes" or 0 for "No"
23d	Are there protocols and guidelines for diagnosing pregnancy in adolescent clients?	0=No 1=Yes	Score 1 for "Yes" or 0 for "No"
23e	Are there protocols and guidelines for treating STIs/RTIs in adolescent clients?	0=No 1=Yes	Score 1 for "Yes" or 0 for "No"
23f	Are there protocols and guidelines for providing care to adolescent clients during their pregnancy?	0=No 1=Yes	Score 1 for "Yes" or 0 for "No"
23g	Are there protocols and guidelines for providing care to adolescent clients during their childbirth?	0=No 1=Yes	Score 1 for "Yes" or 0 for "No"
23h	Are there protocols and guidelines for providing care to adolescent clients after their childbirth?	0=No 1=Yes	Score 1 for "Yes" or 0 for "No"
23i	Are there protocols and guidelines for providing abortion services to adolescent clients (where they are legal)?	0=No 1=Yes	Score 1 for "Yes" or 0 for "No"

Continues...

Continued from previous page

No.	Question	Response	Score
23j	Are there protocols and guidelines for information and counselling on contraception, including emergency contraception, to adolescent clients?	0=No 1=Yes	Score 1 for "Yes" or 0 for "No"
23k	Are there protocols and guidelines for providing information and counselling on condoms to adolescent clients?	0=No 1=Yes	Score 1 for "Yes" or 0 for "No"
23l	Are there protocols and guidelines for providing care and support to HIV-positive adolescents?	0=No 1=Yes	Score 1 for "Yes" or 0 for "No"
23m	Are there protocols and guidelines for providing care and support to adolescent clients who have been physically or sexually assaulted?	0=No 1=Yes	Score 1 for "Yes" or 0 for "No"
	Aggregate observation score		**Total score**

Overall score on Characteristic 18

	Category	Min – Max	Score
1	**Aggregate health-care provider score**	0 – 13	
2	**Aggregate manager score**	0 – 13	
3	**Aggregate observation score**	0 – 13	
	Absolute total score	0 – 39	
	Relative score for Characteristic 18	0 to 100%	$\left(\frac{\text{Total score}}{39}\right) \times 100$

CHARACTERISTIC 19

Health-care providers are able to dedicate sufficient time to work effectively with their adolescent clients

It's a long story; I don't know where to begin.
It's OK, just take your time and tell me when you are ready.

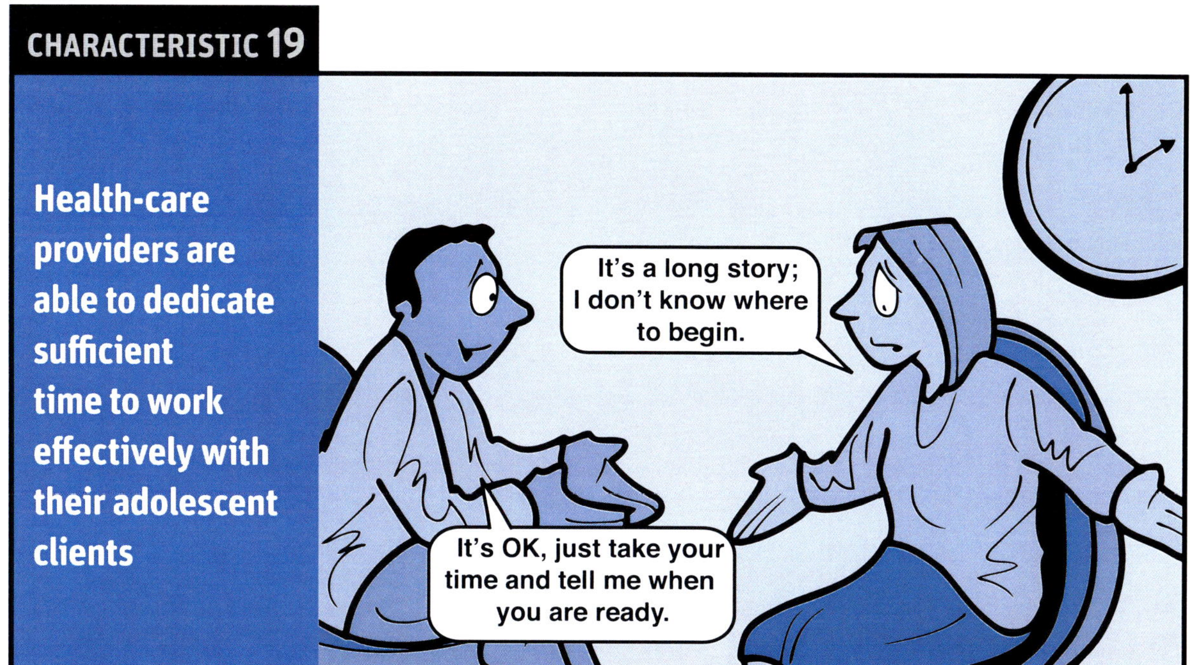

Adolescent client tool:

No.	Question	Response	Score
46	Did you have enough time to ask the health-care provider everything you wanted to ask?	0=No 1=Yes	Total "Yes" divided by total number of adolescent clients interviewed
47	Did the health-care provider answer your questions in a relaxed manner or did he/she seem rushed and hurried to see the next client?	0=No 1=Yes	Total "Yes" divided by total number of adolescent clients interviewed
	Aggregate adolescent client score		**Total score**

Health-care provider tool:

No.	Question	Response	Score
21	In your opinion, do you have enough time for your consultations with your adolescent clients?	0=No 1=Yes	Total "Yes" divided by total number of health-care providers interviewed
22	Do you sometimes have to see your clients quickly because there are many clients waiting to see you?	0=Yes 1=No	Total "No" divided by total number of health-care providers interviewed
	Aggregate health-care provider score		**Total score**

Overall score on Characteristic 19

	Category	Min – Max	Score
1	**Aggregate adolescent client score**	0 – 2	
2	**Aggregate health-care provider score**	0 – 2	
	Absolute total score	0 – 4	
	Relative score for Characteristic 19	0 to 100%	$\left(\frac{\text{Total score}}{4}\right) \times 100$

SCORING SHEETS

CHARACTERISTIC 20

The point of health service delivery has the required equipment, supplies, and basic services necessary to deliver the required health services

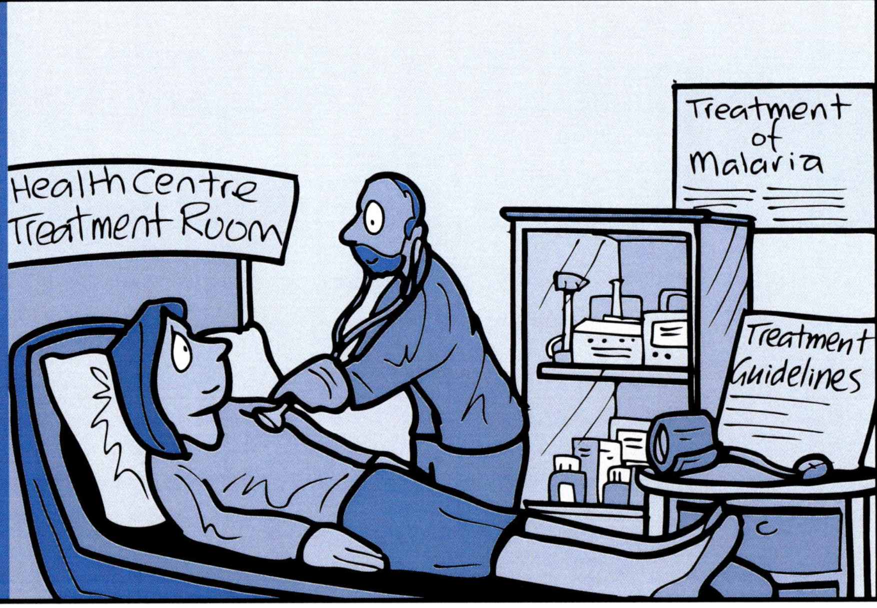

Adolescent client tool:

No.	Question	Response	Score
48	Did the health facility have all the medicines and supplies needed to deal with your needs?	0=No 1=Yes	Total "Yes" divided by total number of adolescent clients interviewed
	Aggregate adolescent client score		**Total score**

Health-care provider tool:

No.	Question	Response	Score
23	Do you have all the medicines and supplies you need to manage your patients?	0=No 1=Yes	Total "Yes" divided by total number of health-care providers interviewed
24	In the last six months, have you had shortages or stock-outs of medicines and supplies that disrupted the provision of services offered?	0=Yes 1=No	Total "No" divided by total number of health-care providers interviewed
25	Do you have all the equipment you need to manage your patients?	0=No 1=Yes	Total "Yes" divided by total number of health-care providers interviewed
26	In the last six months, has unavailability of equipment or non-functioning equipment disrupted the provision of services offered?	0=Yes 1=No	Total "No" divided by total number of health-care providers interviewed
	Aggregate health-care provider score		**Total score**

Manager tool:

No.	Question	Response	Score
21	Does the health facility have a system for maintaining an inventory and recording the amount of medicines and supplies in stock?	0=No 1=Yes	Score 1 for "No" or 0 for "Yes"
22	In the last six months, have you had shortages or stock-outs of medicines and supplies that disrupted the provision of any services offered?	0=Yes 1=No	Score 1 for "No" or 0 for "Yes"
23	In the last six months, has unavailability of equipment or non-functioning equipment disrupted the provision of services offered?	0=Yes 1=No	Score 1 for "No" or 0 for "Yes"
	Aggregate manager score		**Total score**

Observation guide:

No.	Question	Response	Score
24	Does the health facility have a system for maintaining an inventory and recording the amount of medicines and supplies in stock?	0=No 1=Yes	Score 1 for "Yes" or 0 for "No"
25	Does the health facility have the required basic equipment necessary to deliver the essential care package?	0=No 1=Yes	Score 1 for "No" or 0 for "Yes"
	Aggregate observation score		**Total score**

SCORING SHEETS

Overall score on Characteristic 20

	Category	Min – Max	Score
1	**Aggregate adolescent client score**	0 – 1	
2	**Aggregate health-care provider score**	0 – 4	
3	**Aggregate manager score**	0 – 3	
4	**Aggregate observation score**	0 – 2	
	Absolute total score	0 – 10	
	Relative score for Characteristic 20	0 to 100%	$\left(\frac{\text{Total score}}{10}\right) \times 100$

Instruments for data collection

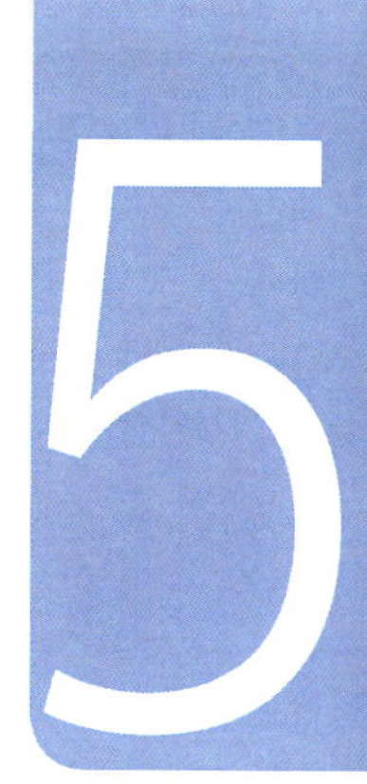

Adolescent client interview tool

Method:

Use this tool to collect information from approximately six adolescent clients who received a reproductive health service at a health facility. Select a private location away from the health facility and explain to the adolescent clients that their names will not be used or recorded and that all the information they provide will be confidential. You can use the greeting below to introduce yourself and the purpose for talking with them:

Greeting:

Hello. My name is ________________ and I work for the ________________. I would like to talk to you about your experience of using this health facility. I am interested in your opinions because we are trying to find out how adolescents feel about getting reproductive health services at this health facility. I would like to ask you a few questions that should not take more than 30 minutes. I will not write down your name and everything you tell me will be kept strictly confidential. You do not have to participate in this interview, and if you do choose to be interviewed, you do not have to answer every question I ask you. Do you have any questions about this?

Demographics:

1. Sex of client (note but do not ask)
2. What is your age?
3. Are you currently studying (in school, college or elsewhere)?
4. What is the highest level of education that you have completed?
5. What is your marital status?

Adolescent-friendly health service characteristics:

Policies and procedures are in place that do not restrict the provision of health services on any terms

6. Have you ever come to this health facility and not been able to receive a particular type of health service?
   a. If so, do you know why you could not receive the health service?
7. Are any health services offered at this facility that you think some groups of adolescents might not be able to receive?
   a. If so, explain which health services and what groups of adolescents.
   b. Why do you think that such an adolescent might not receive that health service(s)?

Health-care providers treat all adolescent clients with equal care and respect, regardless of status

8. Has the health-care provider treated you in a manner that made you feel respected?

9. Did the health-care provider make you feel comfortable?

Support staff treat all adolescent clients with equal care and respect, regardless of status

10. Has the receptionist treated you in a manner in which you would want to be treated?
11. Did the receptionist make you feel comfortable?
12. Have other support staff, such as security staff, clerical staff and cleaning staff, treated you in a manner in which you would want to be treated?
13. Did the other support staff, such as security staff, clerical staff and cleaning staff, make you feel comfortable?

Policies and procedures are in place that ensure that health services are either free or affordable to adolescents

14. Were you asked to pay for health services?
    a. If you were asked to pay for health services, were you able to pay?
    b. In case you could not pay, did you receive the health services anyway?

The point of health service delivery has convenient hours of operation

15. Do you know the days and times that the health facility is open?
16. Are the working days and working hours of the health facility convenient for you?

Adolescents are well-informed about the range of available reproductive health services and how to obtain them

17. Could you tell me which reproductive health services are offered at this health facility?
18. How did you hear/learn about this?

Community members understand the benefits that adolescents will gain by obtaining the health services they need, and support their provision

19. Do you think that your parents/guardians would be supportive of you coming to this health facility for reproductive health services?
20. Are there some reproductive health services your parent/guardians might not want to be provided to you?
    a. If so, which ones?
21. Do you think other adults in the community are supportive of adolescents coming to this health facility for reproductive health services?
    a. How do you know this?

Some health services and health-related commodities are provided to adolescents in the community by selected community members, outreach workers and adolescents themselves

22. Are you aware of any health services that are provided to adolescents in the community?
    a. If so, what type of health service is being provided?
    b. Could you tell me who is providing the health service (i.e. a health-care provider from the health facility, an outreach worker or a community member)?

Policies and procedures are in place that guarantee client confidentiality

23. Do you believe that the information you shared with the health-care provider will be kept confidential?
24. Do you believe that the receptionist or other support staff working there will keep your information confidential?
25. Do you think the following is true (yes/no/not sure):
    a. If you tell a doctor something personal, others in the health facility or the community will find out.
    b. If you tell a nurse something personal, others in the health facility or the community will find out.

The point of health service delivery ensures privacy

26. When you visited the health facility, did you believe that other clients could see you and hear you, and know what you came for?
27. When you were talking to the person at the reception/registration counter, could other people hear you?
28. Did anyone interrupt your discussion with the health-care provider?
29. Do you believe that others could hear your discussions with the health-care provider when you were in the consultation/examination/treatment room?

Health-care providers are non-judgmental, considerate, and easy to relate to

30. Did the health-care provider give you his/her full attention?
31. Did the health-care provider seem interested in what you had to say?
32. Did the health-care provider respect your opinion and decisions even if they were different from his or hers?
    a. If so, could you give me an example?
33. Did the health-care provider treat you in a supportive and considerate manner?

The point of health service delivery ensures consultations occur in a short waiting time, with or without an appointment, and (where necessary) swift referral

34. Have you found the waiting times to see the health-care provider reasonable?
35. Did the health-care provider refer you to another place?
    a. If so, did he/she explain to you why you were being referred to another place?
    b. If so, did he/she explain to you where and when to go?

The point of health service delivery has an appealing and clean environment

36. Did you find the health facility a welcoming place to come to?
37. Did you find all areas of the health facility that you used to be clean?
    a. Surroundings?
    b. Reception area?
    c. Waiting room?
    d. Toilets?
    e. Consultation room/examination room?

The point of health service delivery provides information and education through a variety of channels

38. Did you see informational/educational materials on adolescent health topics during your visit to the health facility?
    a. Were the materials useful?
    b. Were they easy to read?
    c. Were they interesting to read?

Adolescents are actively involved in designing, assessing and providing health services

39. Are you aware of adolescents who were/are involved in contributing to decisions about how health services should be delivered to adolescent clients?
    a. If so, what do/did they do?
40. Do you believe that you could make a suggestion to the staff for improving the way in which health services are delivered here? Explain.

The required package of health care is provided to fulfil the needs of all adolescents either at the point of health service delivery or through referral linkages

41. Did you receive the health service you need to deal with your health concern or health problem?
42. Were you referred to another health facility for health services not available at this one?
    b. If so, what did the health-care provider do to ensure that you receive the health services for which you have been referred?

Health-care providers have the required competencies to work with adolescents and to provide them with the required health services

43. Did the health-care provider explain things in a way you could understand?
44. Did the health-care provider explain to you:
    a. what check-ups/tests he or she was doing?
    b. the results of the check-ups/tests?
    c. what treatment he or she was proposing and why?
45. Did the health-care provider:
    a. discuss the pros and cons of the different treatment approaches with you?
    b. ask you which treatment option you preferred?

Health-care providers are able to dedicate sufficient time to work effectively with their adolescent clients

46. Did you have enough time to ask the health-care provider everything you wanted to ask?
47. Did the health-care provider answer your questions in a relaxed manner or did he/she seem rushed and hurried to see the next client?

The point of health service delivery has the required equipment, supplies, and basic services necessary to deliver the required health services

48. Did the health facility have all the medicines and supplies to deal with your needs?

Health-care provider interview tool

Method:

Use this tool to collect information from approximately five health-care providers who provide reproductive health services at a health facility. See the chart in the section on planning for the assessment for more details on ideal sample size. Select a private location away from the health facility and explain to the health-care providers (separately) that their names will not be used or recorded and that all the information they provide will be confidential. You can use the greeting below to introduce yourself and the purpose for talking with them:

Greeting:

Hello. My name is ___________________ and I work for the ___________________. I would like to talk to you about your experience in providing reproductive health services to adolescent clients. I am interested in your opinions because we are trying to find out how health-care providers feel about providing reproductive health services to adolescents at this facility. I would like to ask you a few questions that should not take more than 30 minutes. I will not write down your name and everything you tell me will be kept strictly confidential. You do not have to participate in this interview, and if you do choose to be interviewed, you do not have to answer every question I ask you. Do you have any questions about this?

Demographics:

1. Sex of health-care provider (note but do not ask)
2. How many years have you worked at this facility?
3. What are your areas of responsibility in this facility?
4. Circle the type of health-care provider:
   a. Doctor
   b. Nurse
   c. Nursing assistant
   d. Midwife
   e. Other: ______________________________

Adolescent-friendly health service characteristics:

Policies and procedures are in place that do not restrict the provision of health services on any terms

5. Are there certain policies or procedures at this facility that might restrict the provision of health services to some groups of adolescents, such as those who are less than a certain age; those who are not married; or those who belong to a certain group, such as people living or working on the street?
   a. If so, could you describe what these policies or procedures are?

6. Can you describe the characteristics of some adolescents who may be denied services?

Health-care providers treat all adolescent clients with equal care and respect, regardless of status

7. Are there some groups of adolescents who you do not feel comfortable dealing with (e.g. those less than a certain age, those who are unmarried)?
   b. If so, could you explain why you feel uncomfortable?

Community members understand the benefits that adolescents will gain by obtaining the health services they need, and support their provision

8. Do community members support the provision of reproductive health services to adolescents?
   a. If so, do they assist you in any way? Explain how.

Policies and procedures are in place that guarantee client confidentiality

9. Are there any policies or procedures in place that guarantee the confidentiality of adolescent clients in this health facility?
   a. If so, what specifically do they say?

10. Are there any circumstances in which you would not follow any of these policies or procedures?
    a. If so, could you explain?

The point of health service delivery ensures privacy

11. Are you ever interrupted by other staff when providing services to adolescent clients?
12. Is it possible for other people to hear your conversations or counselling sessions with adolescent clients?

The point of health service delivery ensures consultations occur in a short waiting time, with or without an appointment, and (where necessary) swift referral

13. Do you know the procedures for making referrals for adolescent clients?
    a. If so, could you describe them to me?

14. Are adolescent clients provided with any assistance with the referral?

The required package of health care is provided to fulfil the needs of all adolescents either at the point of health service delivery or through referral linkages

15. Are adolescent clients offered the following reproductive health services?
    a. Information and counselling on reproductive health, sexuality and safe sex
    b. Testing and counselling services for HIV
    c. STI/RTI diagnosis
    d. Pregnancy diagnosis
    e. Treatment for STIs/RTIs
    f. Care during pregnancy
    g. Care during childbirth
    h. Care after childbirth
    i. Abortion services (where they are legal)

j. Information and counselling on contraception, including emergency contraception
k. Information and counselling on condoms
l. Care and support to HIV-positive adolescents
m. Care and support to adolescent clients who have been physically or sexually assaulted

16. If some services are not available at your health facility, do you know how and where to refer clients for these services?

Health-care providers have the required competencies to work with adolescents and to provide them with the required health services

17. Do you believe that you have adequate knowledge and skills to provide health services to adolescent clients in the following areas?
    a. Information and counselling on reproductive health, sexuality and safe sex
    b. Testing and counselling services for HIV
    c. STI/RTI diagnosis
    d. Pregnancy diagnosis
    e. Treatment for STIs/RTIs
    f. Care during pregnancy
    g. Care during childbirth
    h. Care after childbirth
    i. Abortion services (where they are legal)
    j. Information and counselling on contraception, including emergency contraception
    k. Information and counselling on condoms
    l. Care and support to HIV-positive adolescents
    m. Care and support to adolescent clients who have been physically or sexually assaulted

18. Do you believe that you are able/trained to communicate with adolescents about the risks, benefits and potential complications of the treatments and procedures you provide?
19. Do you tell adolescent clients about alternatives to such procedures/treatments?

Health-care providers use evidence-based protocols and guidelines to provide health services

20. Please indicate whether you use protocols and guidelines at your health facility for the following health services:
    a. Information and counselling on reproductive health, sexuality and safe sex
    b. Testing and counselling services for HIV
    c. STI/RTI diagnosis
    d. Pregnancy diagnosis
    e. Treatment for STIs/RTIs
    f. Care during pregnancy
    g. Care during childbirth
    h. Care after childbirth
    i. Abortion services (where they are legal)
    j. Information and counselling on contraception, including emergency contraception

k. Information and counselling on condoms

l. Care and support to HIV-positive adolescents

m. Care and support to adolescent clients who have been physically or sexually assaulted

Health-care providers are able to dedicate sufficient time to work effectively with their adolescent clients

21. In your opinion, do you think you have enough time for your consultations with your adolescent clients?
22. Do you sometimes have to see your clients quickly because there are many clients waiting to see you?

The point of health service delivery has the required equipment, supplies, and basic services necessary to deliver the required health services

23. Do you have all the medicines and supplies you need to manage your patients?
24. In the last six months, have you had shortages or stock-outs of medicines supplies that disrupted the provision of any health services offered?

    a. If yes, please list the medicines and supplies.

25. Do you have all the equipment you need to manage your patients?
26. In the last six months, has unavailability of equipment or non-functioning equipment disrupted the provision of any health services offered?

    a. If yes, please list this equipment.

Support staff interview tool

Method:

Use this tool to collect information from approximately three support staff at a health facility, including the receptionist. The other two support staff could be identified by asking the manager which other support staff would likely have the most contact with adolescent clients at this health facility. Select a private location away from the health facility and explain to the support staff (separately) that their names will not be used or recorded and that all the information they provide will be confidential. You can use the greeting below to introduce yourself and the purpose for talking with them:

Greeting:

Hello. My name is ________________ and I work for the ________________. I would like to talk to you about your experience with adolescent clients coming to this health facility. I am interested in your opinions because we are trying to find out how staff feel about providing health services to adolescents at this facility. I would like to ask you a few questions that should not take more than 10 minutes. I will not write down your name and everything you tell me will be kept strictly confidential. You do not have to participate in this interview, and if you do choose to be interviewed, you do not have to answer every question I ask you. Do you have any questions about this?

Demographics:

1. Sex of support staff (note but do not ask)
2. How many years have you worked at this facility?
3. What are your areas of responsibility in this facility?
4. Circle the type of support staff:
   a. Receptionist
   b. Security
   c. Other clerical
   d. Cleaning
   e. Other: ________________________

Adolescent-friendly health service characteristics:

Support staff treat all adolescent clients with equal care and respect, regardless of status

5. Are there some groups of adolescents who you do not feel comfortable dealing with (e.g. being less than a certain age, being unmarried)?
   a. If so, could you explain why you feel uncomfortable?

The point of health service delivery ensures consultations occur in a short waiting time, with or without an appointment, and (where necessary) swift referral

6. How long do clients have to wait before they see a health-care provider?
7. Do you know the procedures for making referrals for adolescent clients?
   a. Could you explain?
8. Are adolescent clients provided with any assistance with the referral?
9. Is there anything else that you think should be improved at this health facility to help make adolescent clients feel more welcomed?

Health facility manager interview tool

Method:

Use this tool to collect information from the manager of each facility that you are going to assess. You can use the greeting below to introduce yourself and the purpose for talking with them:

Greeting:

Hello. My name is ___________________ and I work for the ___________________. I would like to talk to you about your experience with adolescent clients coming to this health facility. I am interested in your opinions because we are trying to find out whether this facility is providing the reproductive health services that adolescents need. I would like to ask you a few questions that should not take more than 30 minutes. I will not write down your name and everything you tell me will be kept strictly confidential. You do not have to participate in this interview, and if you do choose to be interviewed, you do not have to answer every question I ask you. Do you have any questions about this?

Demographics:

1. Sex of health facility manager (note but do not ask)
2. How many years have you been a manager at this facility?

Adolescent-friendly health service characteristics:

Policies and procedures are in place that do not restrict the provision of health services on any terms

3. Are there certain policies or procedures at this facility that might restrict the provision of health services to some adolescents, such as those who are less than a certain age; those who are not married; or those who belong to a certain group, such as people living or working on the street?
   a. If so, could you describe what these policies or procedures are?
4. Can you describe the characteristics of some adolescents who may be denied services?

Policies and procedures are in place that ensure that health services are either free or affordable to adolescents

5. Are adolescents charged for specific health services at this facility?
   a. If yes, please give us a list of the health services provided and the charges for each
6. Are fees for adolescent clients less than fees for adult clients?
7. Do you provide concessions for clients who cannot afford to pay for health services?

The point of health service delivery has convenient hours of operation

8. What are the working days and working hours of the health facility?
9. Are the working days and working hours of the health facility convenient for adolescents?

Some health services and health-related commodities are provided to adolescents in the community by selected community members, outreach workers and adolescents themselves

10. Do you provide any type of health services to adolescents in the community?
    a. If so, could you describe what you or your health facility staff do?
    b. Are adolescents involved in any of these activities?
        i. If so, could you describe what they do?

Policies and procedures are in place that guarantee client confidentiality

11. Are there any policies and procedures that guarantee the confidentiality of clients in this health facility?
    a. If so, could you describe what they are?
12. How do you ensure that these policies and procedures are applied?

The point of health service delivery ensures privacy

13. Are there guidelines in place to provide privacy for adolescent clients?

The point of health service delivery provides information and education through a variety of channels

14. Are there informational and educational materials available for adolescents in the waiting room?
    a. If so, could you tell me what is there?

Adolescents are actively involved in designing, assessing and providing health services

15. Do you give adolescents opportunities to suggest/recommend changes to make services more responsive to adolescent clients?
    a. If so, could you describe these opportunities?
16. In addition to being consulted as clients, are adolescents currently involved in decision-making about how health care services are delivered to adolescents?
    a. If so, how are they involved?

The required package of health care is provided to fulfil the needs of all adolescents either at the point of health service delivery or through referral linkages

17. Are adolescent clients offered the following reproductive health services?
    a. Information and counselling on reproductive health, sexuality and safe sex
    b. Testing and counselling services for HIV
    c. STI/RTI diagnosis
    d. Pregnancy diagnosis
    e. Treatment for STIs/RTIs
    f. Care during pregnancy

g. Care during childbirth

h. Care after childbirth

i. Abortion services (where they are legal)

j. Information and counselling on contraception, including emergency contraception

k. Information and counselling condoms

l. Care and support for HIV-positive adolescents

m. Care and support for adolescent clients who have been physically or sexually assaulted

18. If some services are not available, do your staff know how and where to refer clients for these services?

Health-care providers have the required competencies to work with adolescents and to provide them with the required health services

19. Do your staff have the knowledge and skills to provide the following services to adolescents?

    a. Information and counselling on reproductive health, sexuality and safe sex

    b. Testing and counselling services for HIV

    c. STI/RTI diagnosis

    d. Pregnancy diagnosis

    e. Treatment for STIs/RTIs

    f. Care during pregnancy

    g. Care during childbirth

    h. Care after childbirth

    i. Abortion services (where they are legal)

    j. Information and counselling on contraception, including emergency contraception

    k. Information and counselling on condoms

    l. Care and support for HIV-positive adolescents

    m. Care and support for adolescent clients who have been physically or sexually assaulted

Health-care providers use evidence-based protocols and guidelines to provide health services

20. Do you use protocols and guidelines at your health facility for:

    a. Information and counselling on reproductive health, sexuality and safe sex

    b. Testing and counselling services for HIV

    c. STI/RTI diagnosis

    d. Pregnancy diagnosis

    e. Treatment for STIs/RTIs

    f. Care during pregnancy

    g. Care during childbirth

    h. Care after childbirth

    i. Abortion services (where they are legal)

    j. Information and counselling on contraception, including emergency contraception

    k. Information and counselling on condoms

    l. Care and support for HIV-positive adolescents

    m. Care and support for adolescent clients who have been physically or sexually assaulted

The point of health service delivery has the required equipment, supplies, and basic services necessary to deliver the required health services

21. Does the health facility have a system for maintaining an inventory and recording the amount of medicines and supplies in stock?
22. In the last six months, have you had shortages or stock-outs of medicines and supplies that disrupted the provision of any health services offered?
    a. If yes, please list the medicines and supplies.
23. In the last six months, has unavailability of equipment or non-functioning equipment disrupted the provision of any health services offered?
    a. If yes, please list this equipment

Outreach worker interview tool

Method:

Use this tool to collect information from approximately three to five outreach workers per health facility. Select a private location away from the health facility and explain to the outreach workers (separately) that their names will not be used or recorded and that all the information they provide will be confidential. You can use the greeting below to introduce yourself and the purpose of talking with them:

Greeting:

Hello. My name is ___________________ and I work for the ___________________. I would like to talk to you about your experience doing outreach among adolescents in the community. I am interested in your opinions because we are trying to find out whether this facility is prepared to provide reproductive health services to adolescent clients. I would like to ask you a few questions that should not take more than five minutes. I will not write down your name and everything you tell me will be kept strictly confidential. You do not have to participate in this interview, and if you do choose to be interviewed, you do not have to answer every question I ask you. Do you have any questions about this?

Demographics:

1. Sex of outreach worker (note but do not ask)
2. How many years have you worked for this facility?

Adolescent-friendly health service characteristic:

Some health services and health-related commodities are provided to adolescents in the community by selected community members, outreach workers and adolescents themselves

3. Do you provide any type of health services to adolescents in the community?
   a. If so, could you describe what you do?

4. Are adolescents involved in providing any type of health service to adolescents in the community?
   a. If so, could you describe what they do?

Community member interview tool

Method:

You can use this tool as a focus-group interview guide or as an in-depth interview guide, depending on how many community members you would like to interview. For an in-depth interview, use this tool to collect information from approximately two to three community members with similar characteristics (e.g. mothers of adolescents, fathers of adolescents). For a focus-group discussion, conduct one or two focus-group discussions among community members with similar characteristics (e.g. mothers of adolescents, fathers of adolescents). For either type of interview, select a private location away from the health facility and explain to the community members that their names will not be used or recorded and that all the information they provide will be confidential. You can use the greeting below to introduce yourself and the purpose for talking with them:

Greeting:

Hello. My name is ____________________ and I work for the ____________________. I would like to talk to you about whether you believe adolescents should be provided with reproductive health services at the health facility. I am interested in your opinions because we are trying to find out how this community feels about providing reproductive health services to adolescents. I would like to ask you a few questions that should not take more than 10 minutes (or 30 minutes for a focus group). I will not write down your name and everything you tell me will be kept strictly confidential. You do not have to participate in this interview/focus-group discussion, and if you do choose to be interviewed, you do not have to answer every question I ask you. Do you have any questions about this?

Demographics:

1. Sex of community member (note but do not ask)
2. Do you have any children?
    a. If so, how many children are adolescents (aged between 10 and 19 years)?

Adolescent-friendly health service characteristics:

Community members understand the benefits that adolescents will gain by obtaining the health services they need, and support their provision

3. Do you think that adolescents need reproductive health services?
4. Do you believe that adolescents should be provided with reproductive health services?
5. Do you know the reproductive health services that are available to adolescents at this health facility?

6. Are there certain reproductive health services that adolescents should not receive at this health facility?

   a. If so, which ones and why?

7. What efforts has the health facility made to inform the community about the types of services adolescents need at this health facility?

8. What efforts have been made to inform the community about other aspects of adolescent health and development?

Adolescent-in-community tool

Method:

You can use this tool as a focus-group interview guide or as an in-depth interview guide, depending on how many adolescents you would like to interview. For either case, you need to select adolescents who have not been to the health facility being assessed. To recruit adolescents for a focus group or in-depth interview, go to a place where adolescents spend their free time such as a recreation centre, youth centre, or even a school. Ask potential participants if they have ever been to the health facility of interest. If they haven't, ask them if they are willing to participate in an interview or group discussion about the provision of health services to adolescents. For an in-depth interview, use this tool to collect information from approximately five to 10 adolescents (depending on your time and resources). For a focus-group discussion, conduct one or two focus-group discussions among eight to 10 adolescents (per group). For either interviews or focus-group discussions, select a private location away from the health facility and explain to the adolescents that their names will not be used or recorded and that all the information they provide will be confidential. You can use the greeting below to introduce yourself and the purpose for talking with them:

Greeting:

Hello. My name is ___________________ and I work for the ___________________. I would like to talk to you about how you feel whether adolescents like you should go to the health facility (name of health facility) for reproductive health services (give examples). I would like to ask you a few questions that should not take more than 20 minutes (or 30 minutes for a focus group). I will not write down your name and everything you tell me will be kept strictly confidential. You do not have to participate in this interview/focus-group discussion, and if you do choose to be interviewed, you do not have to answer every question I ask you. Do you have any questions about this?

Adolescent-friendly health service characteristics:

Policies and procedures are in place that do not restrict the provision of health services on any terms

1. Have you or your friends been denied health services at the health facility (name of facility)?
    a. If so, could you tell me for what health service?
    b. Do you know why you were denied?

Health-care providers treat all adolescent clients with equal care and respect, regardless of status

2. Has a health-care provider at the facility treated you or your friends in a manner that made you feel upset?
    a. If so, could you say who did this?
    b. What do you think made that person act in this way?

DATA COLLECTION INSTRUMENTS

Support staff treat all adolescent clients with equal care and respect, regardless of status

3. Has the receptionist or any other type of support staff treated you or your friends in a manner that made you feel upset?
   a. If so, could you say who did this?
   b. What do you think made that person act in this way?

Policies and procedures are in place that ensure that health services are either free or affordable to adolescents

4. Have you or your friends been denied health services at the health facility because you could not pay the fee for the health services?

The point of health service delivery has convenient hours of operation

5. Do you know what days and times the health facility is open?
6. Are the working days and working hours of the health facility convenient for you?
   a. What days and times would be most convenient?

Adolescents are well-informed about the range of available reproductive health services and how to obtain them

7. Do you know what reproductive health services are?
8. Could you tell me which reproductive health services are offered at this health facility?

Community members understand the benefits that adolescents will gain by obtaining the health services they need, and support their provision

9. Do you think your parents/guardians would be supportive of you coming to this health facility for reproductive health services?
10. Are there some health services that your parents/guardians might not want to be provided to you?
    a. If so, which ones?
    b. Why do you think your parents/guardians might not want provided to you?
11. Do you think other adults in the community are supportive of adolescents coming to this health facility for reproductive health services? Explain.

Some health services and health-related commodities are provided to adolescents in the community by selected community members, outreach workers and adolescents themselves

12. Are you aware of any health services that are provided to adolescents in the community?
    a. If so, what are they?
13. Are you aware of any adolescents who are involved in providing health services to other adolescents in the community?
    a. If so, could you describe what they are doing?

Observation guide

Policies and procedures are in place that guarantee client confidentiality

1. Do written policies and procedures exist for protecting client confidentiality?
2. How is confidentiality maintained in terms of registration, record-keeping and disclosure when outsiders ask for information?

The point of health service delivery ensures privacy

3. In the reception area, is it possible to hear the conversations between the receptionist and the adolescent clients?
4. In the waiting area, is it possible to hear the conversations between the receptionist and the adolescent clients?
5. In the consultation/examination/treatment area, is it possible to hear the conversations between other health-care providers and their adolescent clients?
6. What are some of the ways you notice that the staff at the health facility ensure privacy for its clients?

Health-care providers are non-judgemental, considerate and easy to relate to

7. Did the health-care provider give his/her full attention to the client?
8. Did the health-care provider appear interested in what the client was saying?
9. Did the health-care provider show respect for the opinions of the client?
10. Did the health-care provider treat the client in a supportive and considerate manner?

The point of health service delivery ensures consultations occur in a short waiting time, with or without an appointment, and (where necessary) swift referral

11. How long is the waiting time (i.e. the time it takes for a client who registers to see a health-care provider)?
12. Did you hear any complaints from adolescent clients about the waiting time?

The point of health service delivery has an appealing and clean environment

13. Are all areas of the health facility that clients use clean?
    a. Surroundings?
    b. Reception area?
    c. Waiting room?
    d. Toilets?
    e. Consultation room/examination room?
14. Does the waiting room have adequate seating for each waiting client?
15. Does the waiting room have lighting sufficient to read?
16. Is the health facility well-ventilated?

17. Is there safe drinking-water available for adolescent clients?

The point of health service delivery provides information and education through a variety of channels

18. Are there any informational and educational materials that adolescents can read/watch while they are waiting?
19. Are there any signs or posters in the health facility that target adolescents?

Health-care providers have the required competencies to work with adolescents and to provide them with the required health services

20. Did the health-care provider have adequate knowledge and skills to provide health services to adolescents in the following areas?
    a. Information and counselling on reproductive health, sexuality and safe sex
    b. Testing and counselling services for HIV
    c. STI/RTI diagnosis
    d. Pregnancy diagnosis
    e. Treatment for STIs/RTIs
    f. Care during pregnancy
    g. Care during childbirth
    h. Care after childbirth
    i. Abortion services (where they are legal)
    j. Information and counselling on contraception, including emergency contraception
    k. Information and counselling on condoms
    l. Care and support to HIV-positive adolescents
    m. Care and support to adolescent clients who have been physically or sexually assaulted

21. Did the health-care provider communicate with the adolescent client about the following issues?
    a. What check-ups/tests he or she was doing
    b. The results of the check-ups/tests
    c. Treatment he or she was proposing and why (if applicable)

22. Did the health-care provider tell the adolescent client about alternatives to such procedures and treatments (if applicable)?

Health-care providers use evidence-based protocols and guidelines to provide health services

23. At the health facility, are there protocols and guidelines for the following services?
    a. Information and counselling on reproductive health, sexuality and safe sex
    b. Testing and counselling services for HIV
    c. STI/RTI diagnosis
    d. Pregnancy diagnosis
    e. Treatment for STIs/RTIs
    f. Care during pregnancy
    g. Care during childbirth

h. Care after childbirth

i. Abortion services (where they are legal)

j. Information and counselling on contraception, including emergency contraception

k. Information and counselling on condoms

l. Care and support to HIV-positive adolescents

m. Care and support to adolescent clients who have been physically or sexually assaulted

The point of health service delivery has the required equipment, supplies, and basic services necessary to deliver the required health services

24. Does the health facility have a system for maintaining an inventory and recording the amount of medicines and supplies in stock?

25. Does the health facility have the basic equipment and supplies necessary to deliver the package of health services?

Note: More detailed checklists for assessing clinical competencies of health workers on selected marker conditions are provided below, along with a list of equipment, medicines and supplies needed to assess and treat these conditions.

Equipment, medicines and supplies needed to assess and treat selected marker conditions

Selected marker conditions	Equipment, medicines and supplies needed
Testing and counselling of HIV in male and female clients	HIV test kits
Diagnosis of pregnancy/management of unwanted pregnancy	Pregnancy test kits Emergency contraceptive pills Treatment for post-exposure prophylaxis of HIV
Management of penile discharge/pain on urination in male clients	Cefixime 400 mg tablets Azithromycin 1 gm tablets Doxycycline 100 mg tablets
Management of abnormal vaginal discharge in female clients	Cefixime 400 mg tablets Azithromycin 1 gm tablets Doxycycline 100 mg tables Metronidazole 400–500 mg tablets Fluconazole 150 mg tablets/miconazole 200 mg vaginal suppositories/clotimazole 200 mg vaginal suppositories
Management of anaemia in male and female clients	Haemoglobin test kit Iron 220 mg tablets/folic acid 5 mg tablets Abendazole 400 mg tablets/mebendazole 500 mg tablets

Checklists to assess clinical competencies of health workers on selected marker conditions

NB Tick the appropriate box, "Yes" or "No":

	Does the health worker:	Yes	No
8	☐ tell the patient that he is going examine him/her now?	✓	
9	☐ check for signs associated with HIV infection?		

DATA COLLECTION INSTRUMENTS

Could I have HIV?

History taking

	Does the health worker:	Yes	No
1	☐ tell the client that he/she is going to ask some personal questions?		
2	☐ reassure the client that all information provided will be kept confidential?		
3	☐ give the client the time to explain why he/she thinks he/she could be infected with/ have HIV?		
4	☐ ask the client if he/she has had unprotected sex in the last 72 hours?[6]		
5	☐ ask about symptoms associated with HIV infection? • Weight loss • Prolonged diarrhoea, cough or fever • Purple bumps on the skin • White patches in the mouth • Painless swelling in glands		
6	☐ ask about factors which increase the likelihood of infection with HIV? • Do you use a condom every time you have sex? Have you had many sexual partners? Has your partner had other partners? • Have you injected drugs? (Only in settings where this is relevant)		
7	☐ ask about symptoms of STI syndromes? • Genital ulcers • Penile/vaginal discharge • Swelling in the groin • Scrotal pain/swelling		

6 This is in order to assess the need for post-exposure prophylaxis.

Assessment

		Does the health worker:	Yes	No
8	☐	tell the patient that he is going examine him/her now?		
9	☐	check for signs associated with HIV infections? • Weight loss of more than 10% • Kaposi lesions on the skin • Fungal infection in the mouth • Generalized lymphadenopathy • Serious infection		
10	☐	check for signs of STI syndromes? • Genital ulcers • Penile/vaginal discharge • Swelling in groin • Scrotal swelling		

Classification

		Does the health worker:	Yes	No
11	☐	correctly classify the adolescent as • **having possible HIV infection – causing symptoms, signs or illnesses commonly associated with HIV infection?** The presence of any symptom or sign associated with HIV infection or any illness associated with HIV infection • **at risk of HIV infection?** The presence of any risk factor for HIV infection, no symptoms or signs associated with HIV infection and no illness associated with HIV infection • **unlikely to have HIV infection?** No risk factor for HIV infection, no symptoms or signs associated with HIV infection and no illness associated with HIV infection		
12	☐	explain the classification?		

Management

		Does the health worker:	Yes	No
13	☐	appropriately manage the adolescent based on classification? • **Having possible HIV infection causing symptoms, signs or illnesses commonly associated with HIV infection** HIV testing and counselling on site or through referral, counselling on safer sex/ HIV risk reduction, treatment of any HIV-related illness • **At risk for HIV infection** The presence of any risk factor for HIV infection, no symptoms or signs associated with HIV infection and no illness associated with HIV infection. • **HIV infection unlikely** HIV testing and counselling, counselling on safer sex/HIV risk reduction		

Counselling & follow-up

		For a client offered an HIV test Does the health worker:	Yes	No
14	☐	appropriately explain • what an HIV test is? • what a positive/negative result means? • why an HIV test should be considered? • that confidentiality will be ensured and that care and support would be provided in case the test is positive?		
15	☐	check the adolescent's understanding?		

Could I be pregnant?

History taking

	Does the health worker:	Yes	No
1	☐ tell the client that he/she is going to ask some personal questions?		
2	☐ reassure the client that all information provided will be kept confidential?		
3	☐ give the client the time to explain why she thinks she could be pregnant?		
4.1	☐ confirm if the client has had vaginal sexual intercourse? (if not already mentioned by the client)		
4.2	☐ ask the client if she was using a contraceptive method correctly and consistently? (if not already mentioned by the client)		
5	☐ ask the client whether her periods were delayed (if not already mentioned by the client) and if she has symptoms of pregnancy? • Nausea or vomiting in the morning • Swelling or soreness in breasts		

Examination

	Does the health worker:	Yes	No
6	☐ tell the client that he/she is going to examine her now?		
7	☐ check for a palpable uterus in the lower abdomen? (if the client is sexually active and could be pregnant)		
8	☐ do a pregnancy test (if available) or refer the client? (if the client is sexually active and could be pregnant)		
9	☐ check for enlarged uterus? (if the pregnancy test is not available and the uterus not palpable abdominally)		
10	☐ check for signs of STI syndromes? • Genital sores/ulcer • Penile/vaginal discharge • Groin swelling • Scrotal swelling (if applicable)		

Classification

	Does the health worker:	Yes	No
11	☐ correctly classify as • **pregnant?** Uterus enlarged on abdominal *or* vaginal examination or pregnancy test positive • **unprotected sexual intercourse within the last five days?** Sexual intercourse within the last five days *and* contraception not adequate *and* NOT classified as pregnant • **unprotected sexual intercourse since the last period, but not within the last five days?** Sexual intercourse since last period, but not within the last five days *and* contraception not adequate *and* less than one month since last period *and* NOT classified as pregnant • **unprotected sexual intercourse with symptoms of pregnancy but too early to be certain?** Sexual intercourse since last period, but not within the last five days *and* contraception not adequate *and* symptoms of pregnancy present, but the uterus is not clearly enlarged, and pregnancy test is not available • **pregnancy unlikely?** Using contraception appropriately and consistently and no symptoms or signs of pregnancy • **not pregnant?** Not sexually active		
12	☐ explain the classification?		

DATA COLLECTION INSTRUMENTS

Management

	Does the health worker:	Yes	No
13	☐ **appropriately manage the client based on classification?** • **Pregnant** – Following counselling, provide antenatal care or abortion services (where they are legal) as appropriate or refer • **Unprotected sexual intercourse within the last five days** – Counsel regarding the risk of possible pregnancy – Counsel regarding options – As appropriate: arrange for review in four weeks to determine whether she is pregnant *or* provide emergency contraception (levonorgestrel 1.5 mg in single dose or ethinylestradiol/levonorgestrel (100 mcg/0.5 mg), two doses 12 hours apart (remember post-exposure prophylaxis to prevent HIV where appropriate) • **Unprotected sexual intercourse since the last period, but not within the last five days** – Advise that although there are no signs of pregnancy it is too early to say definitely whether she is pregnant or not. Discuss future contraception needs and advice. If she does not want to become pregnant, advise her to abstain from sex or use condoms until it is determined whether she is pregnant or not. • **Unprotected sexual intercourse with symptoms of pregnancy but too early to be certain** – Counsel regarding likelihood of pregnancy. If possible, refer her for pregnancy testing. If referral is not possible, discuss future contraception needs and advice. If she does not want to become pregnant, advise her to abstain from sex or use condoms until it is determined whether she is pregnant or not. • **Pregnancy unlikely** – Discuss future contraception needs and advice • **Not pregnant** – Discuss future contraception needs and advice		

Counselling & follow-up

	Does the health worker:	Yes	No
14	☐ appropriately explain • what the condition is? • what the causes of this condition are? • what follow up is needed? – **Pregnant** In line with the algorithm 'I am pregnant' – **Unprotected sexual intercourse within the last five days** Review in four weeks to assess outcome of possible pregnancy – **Unprotected sexual intercourse since the last period, but not within the last five days** Follow up every four weeks for 12 weeks or until it is obvious whether she is pregnant or not If she is pregnant, manage as above – **Unprotected sexual intercourse with symptoms of pregnancy but too early to be certain** Review in four weeks to assess possible pregnancy – **Pregnancy unlikely** As needed for contraception – **Not pregnant** As needed for contraception		
15	☐ check the adolescent's understanding?		

I have discharge from my penis/pain on urination

History taking

	Does the health worker:	Yes	No
1	☐ tell the client that he/she is going to ask some personal questions?		
2	☐ reassure the client that all information provided will be kept confidential?		
3	☐ ask for the nature of urethral discharge? *(if the information has not already been provided by the client)* • Do you have discharge from the tip of your penis? • Do you have discharge from under the foreskin?		
4	☐ ask for symptoms of other STI syndromes? • Genital ulcers • Swelling in the groin • Scrotal pain/swelling		

Examination

	Does the health worker:	Yes	No
5	☐ tell the client that he/she is going to examine him now?		
6	☐ look for • discharge from opening of the urethra? • discharge from under the foreskin?		
7	☐ check for discharge *(if it is not spontaneously visible)* by asking the client to gently squeeze the penis, pressing towards the tip? *(or squeezing it him/herself if the client permits)*		
8	☐ check for signs of STI syndromes? • Genital ulcers • Swelling in the groin • Scrotal pain/swelling		

Classification

	Does the health worker:	Yes	No
9	☐ correctly classify the condition based on symptoms and signs as • **probable STI?** – Gonorrhoea – Chlamydia • **normal?**		
10	☐ explain the classification?		

Management	Does the health worker:		Yes	No
	11	☐ appropriately manage the client based on the classification? • Probable STI: – Treat gonorrhoea with cefixime 400 mg as a single dose orally and – Chlamydia with azithromycin 1 mg as a single dose orally (or doxycyline 100 mg twice daily orally for 7 days) • Normal: – Reassure the client (and if there is discharge from under the foreskin advise regarding hygiene)		

Counselling & follow-up	Does the health worker:		Yes	No
	12	☐ appropriately explain • what the condition is? • what the causes of this condition are? • what the effects of the condition on the body are? • what treatments we are proposing and why? • what the client could do?		
	13	☐ ask the client • to return in one week if symptoms persist? • to inform his partner? • finish the treatment even if symptoms disappear?		
	14	☐ propose an HIV test?		
	15	☐ check the adolescent's understanding?		

I have an abnormal discharge from/burning or itching in vagina (for non-pregnant women)

History taking

	Does the health worker:	Yes	No
1	☐ tell the client that he/she is going to ask some personal questions?		
2	☐ reassure the client that all information provided will be kept confidential?		
3	☐ ask about the nature of discharge? *(if information not already provided by client)* • Colour: clear, white or green/grey/yellowish • Consistency: thin, curdy or thick • Odour: bad smell		
	☐ ask about itching or burning sensation in the vagina?		
4	☐ ask about lower abdominal pain? and if present, assess for conditions needing emergency attention? • Missed/overdue period • Recent delivery/abortion/miscarriage • Abnormal vaginal bleeding		
5	☐ assess for risk of gonorrhoea/Chlamydia? • Client believes she has been exposed to STI • Client has a partner with discharge from tip of penis • Client has multiple recent sexual partners • Client is from a population group or comes from an area with known high prevalence[7]		

Examination

	Does the health worker:	Yes	No
6	☐ tell the client that he/she is going to examine her now?		
7	☐ look for • discharge from the vagina? (colour, consistency, odour) • inflammation of the vulva? (redness, swelling or scratch marks)		
8	☐ feel for tenderness in lower abdomen? If there is lower abdominal pain, in order to assess for surgical/ gynaecological risk feel for: • guarding? • rebound tenderness? • abdominal mass?		
9	☐ do a manual vaginal examination, if there is a history of sexual activity? (to check for tenderness on movement of the cervix)		
10	☐ do a vaginal speculum examination, if there is a history of sexual activity ? and check: • the mouth of the cervix for discharge? • the cervix for friability and redness?		

7 This needs to be based on local epidemiology.

	Does the health worker:	Yes	No
11	☐ correctly classify the condition based on symptoms and signs as • **possible emergency needing surgical/gynaecological attention?** – Lower abdominal pain or tenderness and risk of emergency present • **pelvic inflammatory disease (PID), probable gonorrhoea, *Chlamydia*, and/or anaerobic bacteria?** – Abnormal discharge ○ Colour – whitish/yellowish/greyish/greenish *or* ○ Bad odour *or* ○ Consistency thick or curdy *and* – Lower abdominal pain *or* – Cervical motion tenderness present – No risk of emergency present • **cervicitis, probable gonorrhoea or *Chlamydia*, bacterial vaginosis, and trichomoniasis also likely?** – Abnormal discharge (as above) *and* – No lower abdominal pain or cervical motion tenderness present *and* – Cervical discharge or friability present on speculum exam *or* – Risk factors for gonorrhoea/*Chlamydia* present • **vaginitis with probable candidiasis, bacterial vaginosis and trichomoniasis also likely?** – Abnormal discharge (as above) *and* – Vaginal burning/itching or vulvar erythema *and* – No lower abdominal pain or cervical motion tenderness *and* – No cervical discharge or friability present on speculum exam *and* – No risk factors for gonorrhoea/*Chlamydia* present • **vaginitis, probable bacterial vaginosis, probable trichomoniasis?** – Abnormal discharge (as above) *and* – No vaginal burning itching or vulvar erythema *and* – No lower abdominal pain or cervical motion tenderness *and* – No cervical discharge or friability present on speculum exam *and* – No risk factors for gonorrhoea/*Chlamydia* present • **normal vaginal discharge?** – the discharge is clear and consistency is thin *and* – there is no pain, itching or burning in the vagina *and* – the discharge is cyclic *or* – the discharge is presenting in an adolescent who has not started her menstrual periods yet but is pubescent		
12	☐ explain the classification?		

Classification

Management	Does the health worker:	Yes	No
13	☐ appropriately manage based on classification? • **Possible emergency needing surgical/gynaecological attention** – Refer for surgical or gynaecological opinion • **Pelvic inflammatory disease (PID), probable gonorrhoea, *Chlamydia*, and/or anaerobic bacteria** – Treat for gonorrhoea ○ Cefixime 400 mg as a single dose orally – And *Chlamydia* ○ Azythromycin 1 gm as a single dose orally *or* ○ Doxycycline 100 mg twice daily orally for 7 days – And anaerobic bacterial infection ○ Metronidazole 400–500 mg twice daily orally for 14 days • **Cervicitis, probable gonorrhoea or *Chlamydia*, bacterial vaginosis, and trichomoniasis also likely** – Treat for gonorrhoea ○ Cefixime 400 mg as a single dose orally – And *Chlamydia* ○ Azythromycin 1 gm as a single dose orally *or* ○ Doxycycline* 100 mg twice daily orally for 7 days – And bacterial vaginosis and trichomoniasis ○ Metronidazole 2 gm as a single dose or 400–500 mg twice daily orally for 7 days • **Vaginitis, probable candidiasis, bacterial vaginosis and trichomoniasis also likely** – Treat for bacterial vaginosis and trichomoniasis ○ Metronidazole 2 gm as a single dose or 400–500 mg twice daily orally for 7 days – And candidiasis ○ Fluconazole orally 150 mg as a single dose *or* ○ Miconazole 200 mg vaginal suppository *or* ○ Clotrimazole 200 mg placed in the vagina once daily for 3 days • **Vaginitis, probable bacterial vaginosis, and probable trichomoniasis** – Treat for bacterial vaginosis and trichomoniasis ○ Metronidazole 2 gm as a single dose or 400–500 mg twice daily orally for 7 days • **Normal vaginal discharge** – Reassure the client		

Counselling & follow-up	Does the health worker:	Yes	No
14	☐ appropriately explain • what the condition is? • what the causes of the condition are? • what the effects of the condition on the body are? • what treatments are being proposed and why? • what the client could do? • that the client should complete the full course of treatment? • that the client should return if symptoms persist and when?		
15	☐ check the adolescent's understanding?		

I am too pale (anaemia or suspected anaemia)

History taking

	Does the health worker:	Yes	No
1	☐ tell the client that he/she is going to ask some personal questions?		
2	☐ reassure the client that all information provided will be kept confidential?		
3	☐ ask for severity of anaemia? • Do you feel tired all the time? • Do you get short of breath even when you are seated?		
4	☐ ask about symptoms of possible causes of anaemia? • Presence of acute bleeding • Heavy periods • Inadequate/improper diet • Recent pregnancy or currently pregnant • Malaria • Worm infestation • Long-term illness		

Examination

	Does the health worker:	Yes	No
5	☐ tell the client that he/she is going to examine him now?		
6	☐ check for severity of anaemia? • Pallor, count respiratory rate • Breathless when seated • Haemoglobin level (if possible to check)		
7	☐ check for signs of acute bleeding (gums) and does tests if relevant and possible (does a stool test if there is history of blood in stools or black stools)?		
8	☐ check for excessive bruising, petechiae?		

	Does the health worker:	Yes	No
9	☐ correctly classify the condition based on symptoms and signs as • **severe anaemia or other severe problems?** – Haemoglobin less than 7 g/100 ml *or* – Any of the following ○ Respiratory rate more than 30 breaths per minute ○ Breathless when seated ○ Excessive bleeding from the gums ○ Excessive bruising ○ Petechiae ○ Blood in stools/black stool *or* – If haemoglobin testing is not possible: Severe palmar pallor • **mild to moderate anaemia?** – Haemoglobin more than or equal to 7 g/100 ml but less than 12 g/ 100 ml *or* – If haemoglobin testing is not possible: Some palmar or conjunctival pallor and respiratory rate less than 30 breaths per minute *and* ○ No breathlessness when seated ○ No bleeding gums ○ No excessive bruising ○ No petechiae ○ No blood in stools/no black stool • **no anaemia?** – Haemoglobin is more than or equal to 12 g/100 ml *or* – If haemoglobin testing is not possible: No signs or symptoms of anaemia		
10	☐ explain the classification?		

Classification

DATA COLLECTION INSTRUMENTS

Management

Does the health worker:		Yes	No
11	☐ appropriately manage based on classification? • **Severe anaemia or other severe problems** – Refer • **Mild to moderate anaemia** – Treat anaemia ○ Iron-folic acid tablets 200 mg ○ Start one tablet orally three times per day. Gradually increase to three tablets per day if there is no upset stomach ○ Treat for three months – Address diet ○ Discuss ways to improve diet. Advise to eat foods rich in iron and folic acid i.e. green leafy vegetables, sprouted seeds, and meat – Deworm ○ If the adolescent has not taken deworming medication within the last six months, give a single-dose oral therapy of albendazole (400 mg) *or* mebendazole (500 mg) – Manage causal factors ○ Acute bleeding ○ Heavy periods ○ Pregnancy related ○ Recurrent malaria ○ Other illnesses • **No anaemia** – Reassure the adolescent that they are not anaemic – Address all other conditions and concerns elicited even though they may not be causing anaemia		

Counselling & follow-up

Does the health worker:		Yes	No
12	☐ appropriately explain • what the condition is? • what the causes of this condition are? • what the effects of the condition on the body are? • what treatments we are proposing and why? • what the adolescent can do?		
13	☐ explain that the adolescent needs to come back for follow up? • For causal factors as needed • After three months for check of anaemia		